Assistive Technology for Rehabilitation Therapists

Jennifer Angelo, PhD, OTR, FAOTA
Director, Occupational Therapy
Graduate Program
University of Pittsburgh
Pittsburgh, Pennsylvania

Editor
Shelly Lane, PhD, OTR, FAOTA
Associate Professor
Department of Occupational Therapy
State University of New York at Buffalo
Buffalo, New York

F. A. DAVIS COMPANY • Philadelphia

F. A. Davis Company
1915 Arch Street
Philadelphia, PA 19103

Publisher, Allied Health: Jean-François Vilain
Allied Health Editor: Lynn Borders Caldwell
Developmental Editor: Crystal Spraggins
Production Editors: Nancee Vogel and Rose Gabbay
Cover Designer: Louis J. Forgione

As new scientific information becomes available through basic and clinical research, recommended treatments and drug therapies undergo changes. The author and publisher have done everything possible to make this book accurate, up to date, and in accord with accepted standards at the time of publication. The author, editors, and publisher are not responsible for errors or omissions or for consequences from application of the book, and make no warranty, expressed or implied, in regard to the contents of the book. Any practice described in this book should be applied by the reader in accordance with professional standards of care used in regard to the unique circumstances that may apply in each situation. The reader is advised always to check product information (package inserts) for changes and new information regarding dose and contraindications before administering any drug. Caution is especially urged when using new or infrequently ordered drugs.

Library of Congress Cataloging-in-Publication Data

Angelo, Jennifer, 1952–
    Assistive technology for rehabilitation therapists / Jennifer
Angelo ; editor, Shelly J. Lane.
        p.   cm.
    Includes bibliographical references and index.
    ISBN 0-8036-0136-0
    1. Rehabilitation technology.   2. Physically handicapped children—
Rehabilitation.   I. Lane, Shelly J.   II. Title.
    RM950.A53   1996
617′.03—dc20   96-19181

This book is dedicated to my father, who was the first to show me the way.

Eber L. Burgess, OTR (1913–1977)

FOREWORD

Throughout history, humankind has been either driven or guided by technological advances. From the invention of the wheel to the invention of the computer chip, technology has affected and enhanced our lives.

More recently, therapists have begun to appreciate how technology, specifically *assistive technology,* can also enhance not-so-typical lives, offering easier and more efficient means of task accomplishment, as well as access to life opportunities that were not readily available to individuals with disabilities even 10 years ago. This opportunity for life enhancement must be capitalized on, yet it presents an infinite number of challenges for the rehabilitation therapist.

Challenge 1: How Do I Learn the Basics?

Where does one look when faced with the need for assistive technology for a client? How can a child with limited motor control still play? What can be done to offer an adult with limited mobility access to both the television and the computer?

Challenge 2: What Are the Options?

What are the choices that therapists must consider to optimize the client's skills? How does seating and positioning affect an individual's ability to control his or her environment? How will adapted toys affect a child's ability to play? How will adapted computers and environmental control units affect an adult's ability to work?

Challenge 3: Where Is the Best Choice Found, and How Does It Get Funded?

Can the client be served by Medicaid or Medicare? Is private insurance the way to go? Should I force the issue with the school system? What are the pros and cons of these choices?

Challenge 4: How Do I Know When My Client Is Ready for Something New?

If the client is a child, it is unlikely that a single assistive technology intervention will suffice for a lifetime. If the client is an adult, needs may also change with time. Building growth into an initial system is important, but knowing when to change is important too.

Challenge 5: Assistive Technology Seems to Change So Quickly. How Can I Keep Up? Must I Know It All?

What is the basic foundational information that I must know? In what area(s) will I concentrate? In what area(s) do I need to have the latest information at my finger tips? Who are the experts in assistive technology that I can easily call when I have questions regarding particular areas of assistive technology? Are there catalogs, conferences, vendors, websites, and list serves that I can use to help me keep up with the changes?

Assistive Technology for Rehabilitation Therapists does not propose to address all of these challenges, and it is unlikely that any book currently available could do so. What this book does is provide the reader with the basics of assistive technology. Angelo has written, and collected from other experts, materials that address foundational skills in many aspects related to the provision of assistive technology to individuals with disabilities. Angelo and colleagues have addressed computers and augmentative communication; access methods ranging from switches, mice, and trackballs to keyboards; issues related to mounting the device to make it accessible; seating (powered and manual) and mobility; and funding. They have defined a team approach to assistive technology and have taken a lifespan approach to the application of assistive technology. The book is packed with information, and the authors have included case studies to guide the reader in integrating the information into reality. This book provides the reader with an overview of the application of assistive technology, coupled with some specific examples for application. It is at once a great place to start learning and an excellent resource of information for a therapist with a background. *Assistive Technology for Rehabilitation Therapists* is a source of options, ideas, and information as you work to include assistive technology as a therapeutic tool.

Shelly J. Lane

PREFACE

As I began my journey into the area of assistive technology, I started looking for information to guide me. I searched for books, articles, conference proceedings, and workshops for direction. I wanted to understand my role as a therapist. I wanted answers to questions such as: What skills do I already possess that would be helpful? What skills do I need to develop? How would the age, cognitive level, and interest of my clients change how I conducted assessments? The information I needed was difficult to find in written form.

Eventually, abstracts, articles, and books emerged, but these were in some way incomplete. Many abstracts and articles were narrow in scope, covering only a single topic, such as seating options or the effect of seating on hand use. Other articles simply compared one device with another. The books covered a wider range of topics but were written from the perspective of professionals in other disciplines, such as the speech pathologist or the rehabilitation engineer. Some books covered one particular topic but omitted other assistive technology topics. In all of these publications, explanation of the therapist's role seemed to be missing, so the idea for this book developed.

Assistive Technology for Rehabilitation Therapists is practical. It is a concise, yet complete, resource on assistive technology that provides a foundation to therapists inexperienced in delivering assistive technology services. The book should be used as a starting point to provide the reader with a firm foundation in assistive technology without being overwhelming.

This book has been developed specifically with the therapist in mind, but the role of the entire assistive technology team is also considered. The organization of the book will help the reader through an assessment and will help the therapist find answers to such questions as: Who should be on a particular team? What data should be gathered before meeting the client for the first time? What data should be collected at the first assessment and subsequent assessments? How does one start a search for funding? A guide is presented at the beginning of each chapter to help the reader through the process of selecting and implementing the appropriate technology. Case studies presented at the end of each chapter illustrate concepts presented in the text.

It is my hope that this book will be used by students, instructors, clinicians new to the field of assistive technology, and others as they begin their own journey into assistive technology.

Jennifer Angelo

ACKNOWLEDGMENTS

I wish to thank my husband, Hank Weiss, my daughters, Kate and Claire, and my mother for their patience, understanding, and help. Thanks to Elaine Trefler for her idea for the organizational chart and her suggestions in making this book, and to Marsha Saran for giving me lots of opportunities for learning about technology. In addition, I'd like to thank my editors, Shelly Lane and Lynn Borders Caldwell, for their patience and diligence.

I would like to acknowledge the following reviewers. Their comments were most helpful in making this book readable.

Marilyn L. Blaisdell, MA, OTR
Assistant Professor
Occupational Therapy Assisting
 Program
Becker College
Worchester, Massachusetts

Jane Case-Smith, EdD, OTR
Associate Professor
Department of Occupational
 Therapy
Ohio State University
Columbus, Ohio

Cheryl M. Deterding, MA, OTR
Assistant Professor
Department of Occupational
 Therapy Education
School of Allied Health
University of Kansas Medical
 Center
Kansas City, Kansas

Edith C. Fenton, MS, OTR
Professor and Coordinator
Occupational Therapy Assisting
 Program
Becker College
Worcester, Massachusetts

Nancy Whiting Glover, MS, OTR
Lead Occupational Therapist
Charlotte/Mecklenberg Schools
Charlotte, North Carolina

Martha C. Gram, PT
Physical Therapist/Graduate Student
EDSED/University of Illinois at
 Chicago
Department of Physical Therapy
Chicago, Illinois

Mary Lawlor, ScD, OTR, FAOTA
Associate Professor
College of Associated Health
  Professionals
Department of Occupational
  Therapy
University of Illinois at Chicago
Chicago, Illinois

**Aimee J. Luebben, MS, OTR,
  FAOTA**
Director and Assistant Professor
Occupational Therapy Program
University of Southern Indiana
Evansville, Indiana

**Jim McPherson, PhD, OTR,
  FAOTA**
Associate Professor
Department of Occupational
  Therapy
University of Pittsburgh
Pittsburgh, Pennsylvania

**Caroline Ramsey Musselwhite,
  CCC-SLP**
Assistive Technology Specialist
Special Communications
Litchfield Park, Arizona

**Ellen Berger Rainville, MS, OTR,
  FAOTA**
Assistant Professor
Department of Occupational
  Therapy
Springfield College
Springfield, Massachusetts

Pamela Roberts, EdD, PT
Associate Professor
Program in Physical Therapy
University of Connecticut
Storrs, Connecticut

**Elaine Trefler, MEd, OTR,
  FAOTA**
Assistant Professor
Department of Rehabilitation
  Science and Technology
University of Pittsburgh
Pittsburgh, Pennsylvania

Judith C. Vestal, MA, OTR
Associate Professor
Department of Occupational
  Therapy
Louisiana State University
Shreveport, Louisiana

CONTRIBUTORS

Lewis Golinker, Esquire
Director Assistive Technology Law Center
Ithaca, New York

David Kreutz, PT
Coordinator
Seating and Mobility Clinic
Shepherd Center
Atlanta, Georgia

Shelly J. Lane, PhD, OTR, FAOTA
Associate Professor
Department of Occupational Therapy
State University of New York at Buffalo
Buffalo, New York

Susan G. Mistrett, MS, Ed
Department of Occupational Therapy
State University of New York at Buffalo
Buffalo, New York

Susan Johnson Taylor, OTR
Seating and Mobility Specialist
Assistive Technology Center
and
Seating and Mobility Clinic
Shepherd Center
Atlanta, Georgia

CONTENTS

CHAPTER 3
ACCESS METHODS **43**

CHAPTER 4
SWITCHES **71**

CHAPTER 5
LOW-TECHNOLOGY INTERFACE DEVICES 99

CHAPTER 6
POWERED AND MANUAL WHEELCHAIR MOBILITY . 117

Susan Johnson Taylor, OTR, and David Kreutz, PT

CHAPTER 7

WRITTEN AND SPOKEN AUGMENTATIVE COMMUNICATION 159

CHAPTER 8

ENVIRONMENTAL CONTROL UNITS 177

CHAPTER 9

CAN AND SHOULD TECHNOLOGY BE USED AS A TOOL FOR EARLY INTERVENTION? 191

Shelly J. Lane, PhD, OTR, FAOTA, and Susan G. Mistrett, MS, Ed

CHAPTER 10

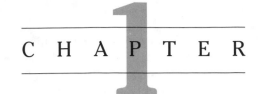

C H A P T E R 1

A GUIDE FOR ASSISTIVE TECHNOLOGY THERAPISTS

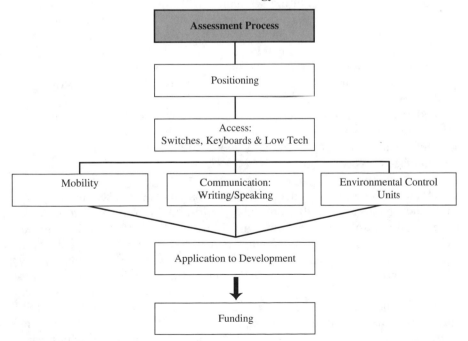

The illustration shown on the previous page will appear at the beginning of each chapter. It organizes the material presented in this book. The content of the illustration that corresponds to each chapter will be highlighted so it is clear where each topic fits. The information in this book is arranged in an order typically used when evaluating persons for assistive technology (AT) devices.

What follows are two scenarios that illustrate how technology can be used with two people at distinctly different developmental levels and with different needs.

SCENARIO 1: RYAN

Ryan is 4 years old, and his mother describes him as "full of life." He smiles and laughs a lot and watches intently as other children run and play. He has favorite television shows (*Power Rangers* and *Shining Time Station*) and favorite foods (blueberry yogurt and macaroni and cheese). Ryan also has cerebral palsy, and this sometimes leads to frustration for his mother and him. Ryan can roll, using his legs and feet to flip himself over when he is prone and using neck extension to initiate the roll pattern when supine. However, this is of limited use when his peers and siblings are running through the house playing *Power Rangers*, so he prefers to sit in his stroller and watch. Because Ryan has only intermittent head control, he cannot always see what is going on, but he joins in the screaming with joy. When *Shining Time Station* ends, Ryan gets frustrated because he wants to change the channel and because he cannot do this independently. He calls for help, but it is not always immediately available. Ryan loves music and, of course, has favorite tapes, but he must rely on others to operate the tape recorder for him. He relies on others to activate all of his toys. Ryan uses his own voice to communicate with his mother; she understands him fairly well. However, Ryan would like to be able to tell his teacher when he feels like eating yogurt and when he would prefer macaroni, but so far she does not fully understand his body language or vocalizations.

Ryan has some obvious needs. He could use specialized seating in something other than a stroller that not only would allow him to have more consistent head control but also would give him the ability to be mobile in his environment and play with his siblings and peers. Proper seating may even give Ryan sufficient upper extremity control to enable him to make a few karate-like moves as a special Power Ranger. Switches in the proper location would provide access so that he could turn the television on or off, change the station, and use a tape recorder. Ryan needs other adaptive devices that will enable independent access to other toys as well. He also needs a communication system that can be activated by access devices that capture his somewhat limited motor control and channels it into choice making and language. The appropriate application of technology could increase Ryan's "developmental level" by 2 to 3 years in a matter of months.

SCENARIO 2: JESSICA

Jessica is about to enter college. She is 21 years old and sustained a head injury 2 years ago, which left her with spastic quadriplegia and limited ability to produce intelligible speech. For transportation, she uses a powered wheelchair fitted with a Jay cushion for pressure management. The back of the chair is a 4-inch piece of foam and a ½-inch piece of plywood that has been upholstered. This back does not provide any contouring to accommodate the curves in the back. The back of her chair encourages flattening of the normal lumbar lordotic curve and accentuates the normal thoracic curve. Jessica is developing kyphosis. A contoured chair back that provides support for the natural curves of the spine may help reduce the kyphosis. To drive, she uses a joystick mounted on the right armrest. She has a portable computer attached to a special lap tray, which was made by her father. The lap tray holds papers for class and her portable computer. She uses the index finger of her right hand to press the keys on the keyboard. Jessica finished high school using this computer. If she speaks slowly, she can be understood by others; however, the listener must know that Jessica is speaking to him or her and move close enough to hear her voice because she cannot produce much volume. Jessica will have other needs as she enters adulthood and is "on her own" at college.

Both of these individuals would benefit from assistive devices to improve their quality of life. For Ryan, such change would affect not only himself but also his entire family and the people involved in his play and educational environments. For Jessica, change includes assuming adult roles and responsibilities. Technology issues that need to be addressed in each of these scenarios include seating and mobility; access methods for control of toys, computers, and other objects in the environment; and functional communication systems. These technology "pieces," when added together and appropriately designed for the individual, support interaction with people and objects within the environment, promote optimal development, facilitate attainment of potential, and improve quality of life for the individual and those within the person's sphere of life. This is the "why" of providing technology.

This book covers the "how" of technology for individuals such as Ryan and Jessica. Technology for seating, access, mobility, environmental controls and interaction, and communication forms the foundation that supports development and fosters independence in individuals with multiple disabilities. The information in this book is organized as one might organize an assessment, except that in an actual assessment, many of the issues would be addressed in quick progression or simultaneously. For clarity, the issues are discussed singly, beginning with seating.

Proper seating can significantly enhance an individual's ability to reach his or her performance potential with other technology devices. For instance, Ryan could be fitted with a head strap for use with his stroller. This would keep his head up consistently and allow him to watch the "goings on" within his environment without interruption. However, most head straps limit head turning and may limit the options available to Ryan for making choices when addressing communication issues. In Jessica's case, a new seating system may be needed to improve posture and to keep her head in a neutral, upright position. Improper seating can result in fatigue, impairing the ability to use assistive devices and to interact with others and the environment. Further, it is imperative to realize that seating, and other technology devices, should be re-evaluated periodically because needs change as the individual develops and grows.

What are the personal mobility needs of the individual? Will a manual wheelchair meet Ryan's needs? Even if he can propel a manual chair, the effort required to do so may be so great that he may have no energy left for activation of an augmentative communication device or computer workstation. This would make manual mobility a poor choice. Is Ryan ready for powered mobility? When the individual being assessed is a child, the team must work with the family and the child. The family may or may not be ready to accept the ramifications of a powered wheelchair, such as the van needed to transport it and the home modifications needed to accommodate the necessary turning space and door widths. The team may need to provide emotional support for the family members as they struggle with the best present mobility solution for the whole family. Presenting powered mobility options may be a long-term goal. In Jessica's situation, these questions might be asked: (1) How old is her present system? (2) What is the terrain like at her new campus? (3) Will her present powered wheelchair be able to keep up with the demands of college, such as traveling from building to building for classes in all weather conditions?

Access is the input device connected to a device. It is the mechanism used to control the device. Keyboards and joysticks are common access equipment. Access is the next logical step in the assessment process. What is the best method of operating an augmentative communication device, a television remote control, or toy for this individual? Does Ryan have more control over his hand, head, or foot? Can he operate a standard or large keyboard? Perhaps a keyboard is not the best solution at all. What about a joystick or a switch? Would a head switch be better once he was properly positioned? Can he activate a large flat switch with his hand or a switch positioned next to his head to play his tape recorder? Does he have more control over his leg than other parts of his body? Can the same movement and input device (e.g., switch, joystick) be used for the tape recorder and an augmentative communication system? These are all access issues, and this list of questions is far from exhaustive. For Jessica, two areas need to be addressed concerning access: the joystick for the power wheelchair and computer access. Is the joystick the best type of input device for Jessica's abilities? Does mounting the joystick to the right armrest make access most efficient, considering Jessica's abilities? Is she able to adequately access the notebook computer keyboard? Does the keyboard placement need to be addressed? What other appliances and tools will she need for access at college? Access may seem a simple area of concern, but it can become complex and intertwined with positioning.

What are the communication and environmental control needs of the individual or the family? Augmentative communication devices will be addressed when reviewing these two individuals' communication needs. Jessica is an excellent speller. Her ability to spell will be considered when recommending augmentative communication systems. Should software be installed in her computer so that it can be used as an augmentative communication device, or should a dedicated unit be recommended? Ryan is ready for simple choice making. Presenting him with two simple selections for choice making would be appropriate as an initial communication tool. Ryan does not yet spell. Should it be assumed that he will learn to spell? His mother understands most of his requests. However, as his experiences outside the home continue to expand, he may have stories to share with his family: He needs communication methods that will enable him to do so. These factors need to be considered as augmentative communication devices are reviewed. Environmental control units allow individuals to control appliances in their environment, such as the television, videocassette recorder, telephone, lights, fan, and radio. Ryan wants to be able to work the television and several toys. How can these needs be met? Seating and access "setups" are significant factors when recommending communication and environmental control systems. How will Ryan's needs change in the future? The need to have a system that is usable at present and allows for growth and development may guide the overall choices. In Jessica's case, some communication training is necessary. Jessica needs to develop strategies for getting people's attention and for speaking as clearly as possible so that unfamiliar listeners can understand her message. She also needs an environmental control unit to control lights, heat, doors, and appliances in her college environment. Ryan needs to be taught basic communication strategies that he can continue to develop as he matures.

This book addresses, in a step-by-step, linear manner, the means by which independence can be fostered with the use of AT in individuals with multiple disabilities. As the reader, you must keep in mind that this linear design will be complicated by application to real people. Case studies on children and adults at the end of each chapter are included to tie the pieces together and reintegrate the information into a whole picture. Chapter 9 addresses the application of technology to the very young child—a group in need of devices and services but frequently overlooked. The last chapter addresses funding. This topic is critical to those involved in the provision of AT devices and services, but it is one about which many of us know very little. The goal in writing this book is to give readers enough information to begin an evaluation for AT needs and to take appropriate steps toward obtaining functional setups for clients.

ASSESSMENT COMPONENTS

Assuming both Ryan and Jessica are referred for assessments of their technology needs, where does one begin? Who will carry out each segment of the assessment? What if you, as a therapist, are the only "technology expert" available at your facility or school? What other input or expertise should you seek out, or can you do the entire assessment yourself? Should you go into the assessment process "cold" to avoid being biased regarding the methods Ryan and Jessica already use? Obviously, there are no absolute answers to these questions, but in the interest of optional assessments for Ryan, Jessica, and other individuals with technology needs, what are the options?

THE ASSESSMENT TEAM

Who are the players in a technology assessment team? The individual with technology needs, Ryan or Jessica, is first and foremost. This individual (and, if the individual is a child, the primary caregiver) will best know his or her own skills, likes and dislikes, and goals for use of technology. As any assessment progresses, Ryan and Jessica, as consumers of the technology, must have the final word on the acceptability of any recommendations.

In some instances, there may be only one other individual involved in the assessment process. This may be a therapist (occupational, physical, speech and language), teacher, or other professional with sufficient knowledge to address the many facets of the technology needs of the individual. Optimally, the team will include two or more of the following, along with the technology consumer and his or her caregiver:

- Seating and positioning specialist
- Interface specialist
- Augmentative communication specialist
- Special educator or educator with additional training
- Rehabilitation engineer
- Funding specialist
- Rehabilitation technology supplier

The roles of these professionals may overlap; thus, the seating and positioning specialist may also function as the rehabilitation engineer, or the interface specialist may also be the funding specialist. Any combination is possible; however, all aspects of the technology needs of the individual must be addressed by knowledgeable individuals.

The Technology Consumer

The needs and desires of the individual come first. If the individual is a child, then the child's parents or guardian and the child need to articulate why they have come for the assessment. If the individual is an adult, the adult (or an advocate) needs to articulate the tasks he or she would like to accomplish independently. The individual's goals may be to improve personal mobility, speaking, or writing, or to write faster. His or her plans may be to attend postsecondary school and use a method of note taking. Perhaps the individual needs a better method of speaking to unfamiliar listeners. He or she may have been working and needs updated computer equipment and software so that he or she can continue to perform the job tasks efficiently. Whatever the desired outcomes, as the assessment progresses, the individual's likes and dislikes of particular types of assistive devices must be considered as recommendations are being made.

Family Members

The family member, guardian, or advocate plays a particularly important role. As noted previously, this person may be the spokesperson for the individual if the individual is unable to describe his or her wants and needs. This individual can also explain the current communication method used with familiar and unfamiliar listeners, the communication system that has been used effectively, and the methods that were tried but were unsuccessful. Similarly, if mobility or environmental control devices are not being used or have been used in the past, this person may be able to contribute invaluable information about the devices and their success or failure. In addition, this individual has knowledge of other influences on the user's life and can assist the therapist in choosing equipment that will best fit into all aspects of the home, school, or work environment.

This person can also help put the individual at ease, particularly a child. This may be the first time the individual is in a room with several strangers who may appear impersonal. The individual and family may have traveled a long distance, and the evaluation environment may seem strange to them. Although the individual will want to do his or her best, the newness of the situation has the potential to interfere with attending to the task and concentrating. Family members can reassure the individual that someone familiar, who knows him or her well, will be staying throughout the evaluation process.

Seating and Positioning Specialist

The seating and positioning specialist has expertise to assess wheelchair seating needs to provide the client with support for motor control and function. The contribution of the seating and positioning specialist is essential for the client's volitional control. With proper seating, the client should be able to maintain a comfortable and functional upright posture. An upright posture provides the necessary foundation for optimally accessing the AT. This team member may be an occupational or physical therapist or rehabilitation engineer.

Interface Specialist

The interface specialist, usually an occupational therapist, determines the body part over which the person has most control for potential access sites. Usually the therapist will observe finger, arm, and head movement followed by the lower limbs. After noting motor control over the limbs, this specialist reviews the advantages and disadvantages of a variety of keyboards, switches, assistive software, and low-technology devices that provide access to computers, augmentative communication devices, environment control units, and other AT devices. At this point, the specialist begins to narrow the choices of the potential input methods that could be recommended. The interface specialist will consult with the seating and position specialist as to the availability of locations on the wheelchair and lap tray for placing keyboards, switches, and mounts. Further, he or she will discuss these options with the augmentative communication specialist to determine what type of communication system may be recommended so that needed input devices can be incorporated into the final recommendations.

Augmentative Communication Specialist

The augmentative communication specialist, most often a speech and language pathologist, is a member of the team when the individual has communication limitations. He or she has knowledge in the area of augmentative communication devices and communication strategies that will improve independent communication.

Special Educator or Educator With Additional Training

The educator can describe the demands placed on the individual in the classroom and the areas related to education with which the individual is having difficulty. Usually, this will be the client's current teacher or one that knows him or her well.

Rehabilitation Engineer

The rehabilitation engineer, usually, but not always, a mechanical or electrical engineer, may contribute to the assessment in the seating and positioning area, or in troubleshooting software when an AT software program will not work with a particular application software program. Additionally, he or she may be called on to fabricate a specialized part needed for the wheelchair, such as a method of attaching a lap tray or specialized mounting device.

Funding Specialist

The funding specialist may be a social worker or other professional who has gained knowledge in the area of funding. Government, private insurance, and creative resources may all be investigated when searching for funding sources.

Rehabilitation Technology Supplier

The role of the rehabilitation technology supplier (vendor) is to supply equipment. Sometimes, suppliers are able to lend equipment for clinical trials and longer-term loans. They can also provide information regarding the latest versions of the devices that they represent. Some are able to assist with funding by working with the funding agencies.

Ryan's case illustrates how a team functions. Of course, Ryan and his parents were team members. They were sent a pre-evaluation form (discussed later in this chapter). This form was used to help compose the team. In addition, the pre-evaluation form helped to alert the team to the need for any consultants. On the form, the family indicated that they wanted Ryan to be able to turn the television on and off independently, play with some toys, and choose foods. They know he may need a power wheelchair, but they are hesitant to discuss it, fearing that if he used one, he would run into the walls and furniture and hurt himself and others.

On the basis of the family's responses on the pre-evaluation form, the following team was assembled:

- **Seating and positioning specialist**—needed to evaluate the possibilities of mounting a seating system to the stroller the family already owned. In addition, he wanted to discuss the possibilities of manual and powered wheelchairs with the family.
- **Interface specialist**—called in to evaluate how Ryan would access any equipment that might be recommended. Additionally, the interface specialist wanted to know what was expected of Ryan at school and what his needs were regarding completing written schoolwork.
- **Augmentative communication specialist**—contacted to work on communication issues. She would evaluate both the immediate need for a simple augmentative communication device and future needs; she also would instruct Ryan's parents on how to repair communication breakdown with Ryan.
- **Funding specialist**—contacted to look for funding sources. She assumed that there may be some resources from the school district. In addition, she knew of a local community group that often sponsored the purchase of equipment for children with particular needs. She also

contacted the parents regarding the type of insurance coverage they had and started collecting the forms that this company used and learn- ing the key words the company looked for when denying and approv- ing claims.

- **Rehabilitation engineer**—asked to work with the seating and posi- tioning specialist to review the possibility of placing a seating system on the current stroller. Additionally, he joined the team to help resolve switch or keyboard mounting issues. The rehabilitation technology supplier was asked to bring a switch and keyboard that the team mem- bers thought they might like to try with Ryan but did not have on hand.

The team requested that Ryan's teacher come to the evaluation. The team wanted a thorough understanding of the expectations for Ryan in that area. If the educator could not come, he or she would be asked to send samples of Ryan's work and the goals for him.

TYPES OF TEAMS

There are different types of teams. The three team models commonly discussed are multidisciplinary, interdisciplinary, and transdisciplinary (Beu- kelman & Mirenda, 1992). In a *multidisciplinary* team, each team member does his or her assessment separately. After the assessments are completed, the team members share the findings with the other team members. Each team member provides the services they have described in their assessment report.

Members of an *interdisciplinary* team also assess clients individually and then meet to discuss the findings. An integrated intervention plan is formu- lated, but each team member retains responsibility for provision of the service they recommend. The team may not meet again unless a problem arises that requires a team-based solution.

In a *transdisciplinary* team, professional lines blur more than in the other two team models. Often the assessment is carried out jointly. After the assessment, the team meets to develop goals and plan intervention. Role exchange may occur at the intervention stage. For example, a teacher may be taught specific therapeutic techniques useful to reduce muscle stiffness and enable greater function from the individual. This in turn might reduce the amount of direct time the therapist would need to be involved with the individual.

Each of the previous models has strengths and weaknesses, and a thor- ough discussion of these is beyond the intent of this book. Regardless of the type of team used, the members need to have mutual respect and trust. Each member needs to be comfortable with his or her own skills and role as a team participant.

PREASSESSMENT INFORMATION

Prior to any portion of the assessment, information needs to be collected so the assessment can run smoothly (Fig. 1–1). Armed with information collected prior to the assessment, the assessment team has a more informed idea of what to expect from the individual in terms of motor and mental capabilities, visual perceptual skills, current methods of communication (written and spoken), computer use, other assistive devices already used, current access methods, and assistive devices that are in use or that have been discarded. As was seen in the Ryan example, collecting this information prior to seeing the individual gives the team the opportunity to make preliminary decisions about which software and access tools to have ready. Software and computer access devices (switches or keyboards) can be set up the day before in preparation for the evaluation. Software can be configured for alternate setups that might be suitable for the strengths and needs of the individual. When the preparation is done well, it can save time. Also, if consultants are needed, they can be contacted in advance to attend the assessment, or a referral can be in process. Collecting information prior to the assessment and adequate preparation reduce the number of visits needed to complete the assessment.

Ryan's case illustrates how and where prior information might be gathered. He may have a recent developmental report in his file. Recent reports from therapies can be invaluable to the assessment team prior to the initial meeting with the client. Therapy reports would include range of motion, present means of communication, hand function, positions that elicit primitive reflexes, and current personal mobility methods. This information may be vital to the technology team in understanding the current motor and cognitive skills, visual perceptual abilities, seating and mobility status, communication, and access methods available to the individual. The team will want to know methods that work and methods that have not worked, aspects of a current system that the individual likes, and factors about technology that frustrate the individual.

The adult with disabilities—and, when possible, the child with disabilities—along with parents, guardians, teacher or job coach, and therapists, should state on the pre-evaluation form their goals for the coming assessment. Additionally, from reviewing the pre-evaluation form, the team can learn the client's and family's expectations and can assist them in being realistic regarding the outcomes. This gives the assessment team an understanding of the expectations involved. Such information can be gathered in written form and, if possible, on videotape.

A videotape can capture the client as he or she engages in various everyday activities. Examples of activities are sitting in a wheelchair, using current locomotion skills (using a wheelchair if appropriate), using the current communication system with someone with whom he or she is familiar, using a computer (if the child uses a computer), and experiencing a typical classroom situation. A videotape of Ryan playing with toys gave the team an idea of

Date_____

Client's Name _____ Medical Diagnosis _____
Address_____ City, State, Zip Code_____
Phone_____
Parent/Guardian's Name_____
AT Therapists_____

1. Reason for Referral:_____
_____
_____

2. Vision   Normal_____ Impaired_____ Blind _____
   Please explain if impaired is checked. _____
_____

3. Has a visual perceptual test been performed? Yes_____ No_____
   If yes, what were the results?_____
_____

4. What education level have you had or what grade are you currently in?_____
_____

5. Please check the box for the services you are currently receiving; indicate whether you are receiving
   the service daily, weekly, or monthly by circling the appropriate word.

Occupational Therapy_____ daily, weekly, monthly   Physical Therapy_____daily, weekly, monthly
Speech & Language Therapy_____ daily, weekly, monthly
Day Programming _____ daily, weekly, monthly   School_____ daily, weekly, monthly
Other_____ daily, weekly, monthly   Sheltered Workshop_____daily, weekly, monthly

6. Is the client influenced by primitive reflexes?
   In what positions is she/he most affected?

7. Please describe the client's present communication skills._____
_____

8. What types of communication systems has the client used in the past?_____
_____

9. What were the problems with the system?_____
_____

10. Please describe the client's present mobility skills._____
_____

11. What types of mobility systems has the client used in the past?_____
_____

12. What were the problems with this system?_____
_____

13. Please describe the client's present computer skills._____
_____

14. What types of computer systems has the client used in the past?_____
_____

15. What were the problems with this system?_____
_____

16. What needs do you want to address at the evaluation?
    A. Communication Needs _____
_____

    B. Mobility Needs _____
_____

    C. Computer Needs _____
_____

17. Is there anything else that would be helpful for the team to know prior to the evaluation? _____
_____

Figure 1–1. Example of a pre-evaluation form.

Videotaping
18. If you have access to a video camera and can videotape the client, please complete the rest of this form and send in the videotape with the completed pre-evaluation form. There are two sessions to tape. Please videotape both if they are appropriate situations for this client. Tape at least 5 minutes of each session.

    A. Communication Session
      1. Tape a close up of the communication system.
      2. Tape the client using his or her communication system in a conversation with another person.

    B. Seating
      1. Tape the client sitting in his or her seating system using a front view and side view.
      2. Tape the client moving in the wheelchair if he or she usually propels himself or herself.
      3. If a lap tray is usually used, place it on the wheelchair.
      4. If the client spends time in other positions (e.g., sitting on the floor, in a chair or in bed), please tape those also.

Figure 1–1. Continued

his positions for play, his engagement by the toy, and what elicits the most attention and interest. What else does he do during a typical day? Where else does he spend his time? A videotape of Ryan in his preschool environment helped the team understand the abilities he needed outside his home environment. Likewise, a videotape of Jessica would provide knowledge of her current wheelchair seating system, her driving skills, and how she accesses her notebook computer.

ASSESSMENT LOCATIONS

Assessments can be conducted in a variety of locations. AT centers can be affiliated with universities, hospitals, and rehabilitation centers. There may be a team consisting of two or more professionals from the list described previously. Public schools also have personnel called technology specialists. Within these facilities, the assessment may take place in a private room, within the classroom, or at different times and locations depending on the needs of the child. At times, all or part of the assessment will be conducted in the client's home or office, particularly when equipment needs to be set up such as a work station. This allows the team to understand the limitation of the home or work environment and the positions in which the client spends a great deal of time. Armed with this information, the team is better equipped to make recommendations that are suitable and harmonious with the environment.

CONCLUSION

With technology, individuals with physical disabilities can perform tasks that they could not without technology. Augmentative communication devices allow children to tell their mothers, "I love you." Ramps, power wheelchairs, and electric door openers allow many people with disabilities to be alone for a few hours and yet provide a route to leave in case of an emergency.

These new abilities allow privacy and the feeling of independence. Other technologies that help provide independence include (1) telephones that can be dialed with a switch instead of a dial pad, (2) telephone headsets that allow people with disabilities to speak privately and allow friends to call for friendly chats, and (3) video arcade–type games and computer games that can be adapted so that children with disabilities can play on an equal level with their able-bodied friends.

Now you have your team assembled and an idea of what you will explore with Ryan and Jessica to promote independence and interaction. The next chapter explores options for technology by looking at clients' positioning for activity and interaction.

STUDY QUESTIONS

1. How do the assistive technology needs of Ryan and Jessica differ? How are they similar? As you ponder these questions, be sure to consider the current strengths and needs of each individual, along with his or her potential for developmental change. How might developmental change impact the choice of assistive technology?
2. Which team members would be essential for Jessica? Would there be others you would add if you could?
3. Consider the models of multidisciplinary, interdisciplinary, and transdisciplinary teams. Which might best suit the strengths and needs of Ryan? Would they be the same for Jessica?

REFERENCES

Beukelman, D., & Mirenda, P. (1992). *Augmentative and alternative communication*. Baltimore: Paul H. Brookes.

Christiansen, C. (1991). Occupational therapy: Intervention for life performance. In C. Christiansen & C. Baum (Eds.), *Occupational therapy: Overcoming human performance deficits*. Thorofare, NJ: Slack.

BIBLIOGRAPHY

Collecting Information Prior to Assessment

State of Florida Department of Education (1988). *A resource manual for the development and evaluation of special programs for exceptional students* (Vol. III-M). Tallahassee, FL: State of Florida, Dept. of Education.

Assessment Tools

Lee, K., & Thomas, D. (1990). *Control of computer-based technology for people with physical disabilities*. Toronto: University of Toronto Press.

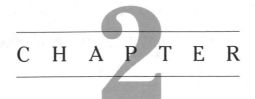

CHAPTER 2

EVALUATION FOR WHEELCHAIR SEATING

Susan Johnson Taylor, OTR

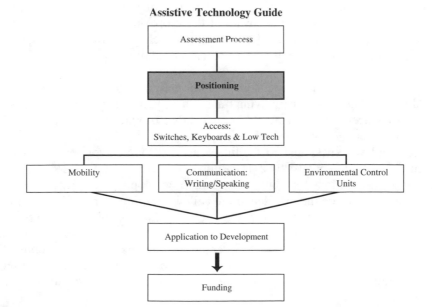

Assistive Technology Guide

```
          Assessment Process
                 │
            ┌─────────┐
            │Positioning│
            └─────────┘
                 │
              Access:
      Switches, Keyboards & Low Tech
       ┌─────────┼─────────┐
   Mobility   Communication:   Environmental Control
              Writing/Speaking       Units
       └─────────┼─────────┘
                 │
        Application to Development
                 │
                 ▼
              Funding
```

THE PURPOSE OF WHEELCHAIR SEATING

Clients with severe neuromotor or neuromuscular disabilities, such as cerebral palsy or muscular dystrophy, are challenging. A large part of a therapist's job is to facilitate the development or maintenance of the client's cognitive, perceptual, social, and motor skills. However, the client who has difficulty obtaining or maintaining positions against gravity will experience delays in these areas. Because of the client's lack of postural control and central stability, he or she experiences a marked decrease in efficiency of movement in attempting functional or activities of daily living (ADL) skills (Colangelo, 1993). Before the occupational therapist can address these skills, the client must be in a position in which he or she is supported and ready to work, play, or learn.

Positioning to be ready to work, play, or learn throughout the day may take on different forms, depending on the age of the client and his or her tasks during the day. For instance, a young child may be positioned in a wheelchair for transport to school or program. If the first program or school activity is circle time and the majority of children are sitting on mats on the floor, then the child with a disability also may be positioned on the floor. If children are standing to play at a water table, this option can be made available to the child with a disability by using a prone stander. Because typical children have many available position options during play and school, the same should be true for the child with a disability. Such seating flexibility for an adult may include use of a scooter for seating and mobility during the day, alternating with use of a wheelchair for other activities that may be too difficult for the scooter or too fatiguing for the adult. This chapter discusses only wheelchair evaluation and seating because of the complexity of these topics. However, you should be aware of these options when planning a program for a client. References at the end of the chapter (Bergen, Presperin, and Tallman, 1990) can guide you in obtaining additional information about other positioning options.

A client who is nonambulatory or minimally ambulatory will probably spend much of his or her daily living time in a powered or manual wheelchair. Inside the wheelchair are external supports that provide the client as much control as is necessary to decrease the effects of gravity, abnormal tone or reflexes, and weakness and to facilitate the development of motor, ADLs, cognitive, and perceptual skills. The supports also accommodate deviations from normal sensations for comfort and inhibit development of pressure sores. These supports inside the wheelchair are called a *seating system*. The external supports in a seating system allow the client to obtain stability in an upright position and receive appropriate, more developmentally normal sensory input, thereby allowing more appropriate interaction with his or her environment. This chapter describes a systematic means to look at posture in the seated position and to provide intervention for a functional outcome for the client.

EXAMINING THE SEATED POSITION

A "neutral" seated position is the ideal goal of a seating system intervention. The pelvis forms the base of support in sitting. The rest of the body responds to how the pelvis is positioned. A neutral pelvic position facilitates the appropriate posture in the client. With a neutral pelvis, the ischial tuberosities bear weight equally, and the anterior superior iliac spines (ASISs) are level from an anterior view (Fig. 2–1). A lateral view will show the anterior and posterior superior iliac spines to be basically level with each other (Fig. 2–2). The trunk is upright with a slight lumbar lordosis. The hips, knees, and feet are at 90-degree angles.

In a person with severe physical disabilities, weakness and abnormal tone and reflexes influence positioning of the pelvis and therefore inhibit the person from obtaining a neutral seated posture. A useful way to experience the effects of various pelvic positions on the body is as follows: Sit on a chair or bench with a flat, firm seat with your feet on the floor with your weight evenly distributed. Now, push your pelvis into a severe posterior pelvic tilt. Note how your body feels. Most likely, your pelvis feels like it wants to slide forward off the chair, and your hips are abducted. Your feet are firmly planted

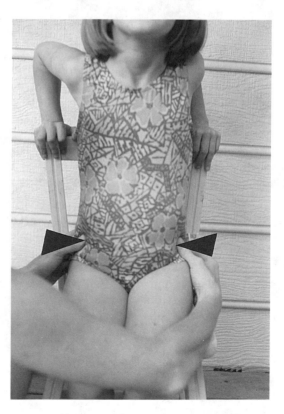

Figure 2–1. The anterior superior iliac spines are level from an anterior view.

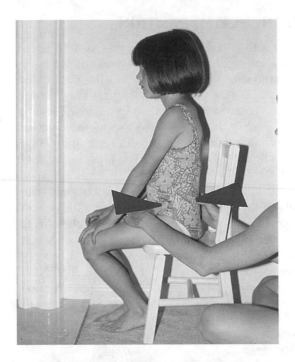

Figure 2–2. A lateral view will show the anterior and posterior superior iliac spines to be basically level with each other.

to prevent further sliding, with more pressure on the ball of the foot than the heel. Your trunk is kyphotic; it is difficult to take a deep breath. Try to reach for something with your left hand across your body to the right side. Because your pelvis is locked in posterior tilt, trunk rotation is nearly impossible. It is difficult to raise your head so your eyes have a level gaze; your neck must hyperextend. Now, imagine how fatiguing this posture is for children who cannot easily move out of it, especially when superimposing the demands of functional skills. This exercise can be repeated with the pelvis in an exaggerated anterior tilt, lateral obliquity, and rotation (Figs. 2–3 and 2–4).

EVALUATION CONSIDERATIONS
The Seating Process and Team Members

Seating should always be considered a *process*. People grow and change rapidly, and the equipment must be able to change with them. As a consequence, seating becomes a process of evaluating, providing equipment, and re-evaluating at regular intervals (Taylor & Trefler, 1984). Careful evaluation of all factors that contribute to obtaining a functional seated posture is required for several reasons. The first and perhaps most important reason is that inappropriate application of seating supports can eventually facilitate poor posture, which can lead to joint deformity. Secondly, this seated posture and the equipment used to obtain it must work in multiple environments and situations, including home, school, and play. Lastly, this equipment is expen-

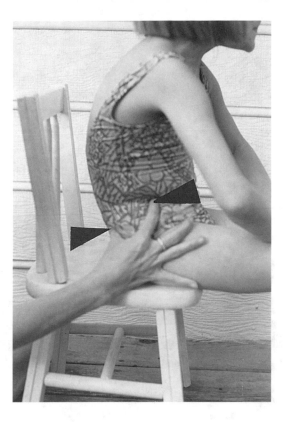

Figure 2–3. A posteriorly tilted pelvis with kyphosis of the spine.

sive, and funding is not always readily available. The team members must work closely with the child and family to ensure that the outcome is functional. In a traditional medical model, the seating team may consist of an occupational therapist, physical therapist, speech pathologist, teacher, orthotist, nurse, physician, and rehabilitation technology supplier (the individual who works with the team to provide the equipment). In today's more fiscally restrictive health care environment, usually just one therapist works with the client and the rehabilitation technology supplier. The therapist becomes the primary information gatherer for the other professionals. The center focus and leaders of the team are the client and caregivers.

The Clinical Framework Used in Seating Evaluation and Provision

As with other therapy, a structured framework for seating evaluation can be followed (Taylor, 1993). Using a framework ensures that a sequence is followed and that all relevant aspects of the child's life are considered in the seating evaluation and provision processes. A sample of such a framework is presented in Appendix A. This framework will be developed below.

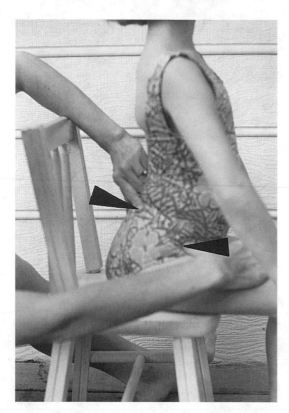

Figure 2–4. An anteriorly tilted pelvis with lordosis of the spine.

Evaluation

An evaluation form is presented in Appendix B to provide a sample outline of the information necessary for a seating evaluation. The evaluation form is set up in the same format as the evaluation section of this chapter.

Information Gathering

The first part of the evaluation consists of information gathering. When a client is being evaluated for seating, one of the first questions the therapist should ask the client and the caregivers (e.g., parents, attendants) is "What are your goals and expectations of this evaluation?" This is because the client and caregivers must live with the equipment. The therapist must determine what is important to the client. With this information, the therapist can keep in mind the client's goals while formulating physical, functional, and ADL goals. The therapist questions the client about his or her present physical, functional, and ADL skills and how these are accomplished. Clients with severe disabilities often already have systems and methods for performing these skills. The therapist observes these skills so that the new seating facilitates rather than interferes with present skills. For example, if the client can transfer in and out of the wheelchair by himself or herself, the therapist would not want to provide a lap belt with the new seating system that the client could not fasten and release independently.

Medical and surgical histories can be influential in the type of positioning provided. Diagnoses must be studied in terms of prognosis and physical or emotional characteristics. For example, clients with diagnoses such as Duchenne muscular dystrophy have a progressive condition that will worsen with age, meaning that their physical and functional needs and abilities will change. Clients with cerebral palsy are prone to joint and spinal contractures because of the abnormal tone they experience. Clients may be medically fragile, such as those who require a respirator or feeding tube (a tube that remains inserted into the abdomen for nourishment and medication). Some clients may have allergies to certain materials, such as certain types of foam or vinyl. All of these types of medically related conditions can have a profound effect on the position in which the child is placed and the materials used to fabricate the seating components.

The therapist must understand what type of surgery the client has had or will be having in the near future that would affect the seated posture. Usually, this is orthopedic surgery, which affects joint or spinal positions or range of motion. For example, a client who has scoliosis (curvature of the spine) may be scheduled to have a spinal stabilization surgery. This would completely change the shape of the spine and therefore change the shape of the back component of his or her seating system.

Physical Evaluation

Neuromotor or Neuromuscular Status

Determining a client's neuromuscular status primarily revolves around observation of movement and clinical assessment of muscle tone and reflexes. It is critical to identify the extent to which these characteristics influence the client's ability to obtain and maintain a seated posture. The therapist must also observe the effects of abnormal tone and reflexes on the client's functional skills and ADL skills. It is crucial that the therapist *feel* these tone and reflex movements, by holding the client on his or her lap or on the examining table. This enables the therapist to feel which positions encourage relaxation in the child or which positions elicit abnormal tone or reflexes. For example, some clients with spinal cord injuries experience spasms of the lower extremities and trunk that are elicited with a change of position, such as moving from sitting to supine.

Clients with neuromotor disorders (cerebral palsy, closed head injury) experience abnormal tone and persistent primitive postural reflexes that interfere with function. Abnormal muscle tone affects the quality or quantity of movement and the ability to grade a muscle contraction. Clients with high tone (hypertonicity), or spastic muscles, generally experience limitations in movement. The hypertonicity is often exhibited in a pattern of flexion, abduction, and external rotation of the upper extremities, with extension, adduction, and internal rotation of the lower extremities (Colangelo, 1993). Clients with low tone, or hypotonicity, are unable to respond quickly to a command to contract a muscle. These people present as "floppy," with very rounded postures. Often, clients exhibit a combination of hypertonicity and hypotonicity. A common pattern is hypertonicity in the extremities, with hypotonicity in the trunk and neck. Athetosis affects the client's ability to perform a graded movement, particularly in midrange. Those with athetosis require a great deal of external stabilization to perform any functional skills.

Primitive postural reflexes are examined with particular emphasis placed on identification of positions or stimuli that elicit the reflexes. Reflexes that particularly affect the seated posture include asymmetric tonic neck reflex (ATNR), symmetric tonic neck reflex (STNR), tonic labyrinthine reflexes, supine and prone (TLRS, TLRP), and the positive supporting reaction. The ATNR and STNR are elicited by movement of the head. With the ATNR, rotation of the head laterally causes increased flexor tone on the skull side with increased extensor tone on the facial side (extremities and trunk). Maintaining the head in midline with a headrest can decrease the effects of this reflex. With the STNR, flexion of the head causes flexion of the upper extremities and extension of the lower extremities, with a rounded back. Extension of the head results in extension of the upper extremities, flexion of the lower extremities, and an exaggerated lordotic position of the trunk. Stable head positioning with a level eye gaze and placement of objects the client must see within the range of level eye gaze usually decrease the effects of the STNR on the client's posture. TLRS and TLRP are elicited by the client's position in space. With TLRS, positioning of the client out of a neutral, upright position (toward supine) with head and trunk in alignment causes an overall increase in extensor tone throughout the body. Conversely, with the TLRP, movement of the head and trunk forward causes an overall increase in flexor tone. Because seating systems often capitalize on tilt in space to provide maximal function and control, the influence this reflex may have on the client's muscle tone must be evaluated carefully.

The positive support reaction is elicited by applying pressure to the ball of the foot. This causes an overall increase in lower extremity extensor tone (extension, internal rotation, adduction). The therapist must consider how the client's foot will be placed and secured on a footrest to avoid eliciting this reflex. Supporting the entire foot with the force of the foot strap over the heel rather than the ball of the foot is one way this can be accomplished.

The therapist's challenge when examining neuromotor or neuromuscular status is one of feeling and understanding the type and intensity of tone and reflexes. Prolonged positioning in these abnormal postures can cause permanent contractures of the joints or spine and can significantly impair function.

Orthopedic Status

The therapist must examine any present contractures or joint or spinal tightness that would inhibit the client from obtaining a neutral seated posture and that must be accommodated by the seating system. When assessing joint tightness, the therapist observes the extent of comfortable joint range and how much force it takes to provide corrective forces. For example, if the client has developed a spinal curvature that is still correctable to some degree with the therapist's hands, the therapist must *feel* how much force it takes to provide that kind of support. Only by feeling the forces necessary to support or correct the deformity can the therapist begin to determine the type of external supports that will be part of the seating system. In some cases, the therapist should refer the client to an orthopedic surgeon to determine whether medical intervention, such as surgery, will help the child to sit comfortably.

The hands-on evaluation, including determination of muscle tone, reflexes, and orthopedic status, is one of the most important steps with which the therapist is involved during the evaluation process. The therapist's "knowledgeable" hands can translate what they are feeling into positions that will facilitate function in the client.

Sensory Status

The therapist must determine areas of impaired or absent sensation. This is of particular concern with clients who have spina bifida or a spinal cord injury and a concomitant absence of sensation. Clients with absent or impaired sensation will require careful attention to the materials of the seating surfaces that contact those areas. Additionally, clients who are thin and bony and are unable to move to shift their weight periodically, such as a client with severe muscular dystrophy or spinal muscular atrophy, also require careful attention to sitting surfaces and materials. For example, seat and back components will have to be made of materials that conform to bony prominences and assist in relieving high pressure around bony areas, which can be prone to pressure sores (e.g., the ischial tuberosities, sacro-coccygeal area, or spinous processes).

Environmental Considerations

The seating system or mobility base needs to function in many different environments. The client functions in the home, at play, and in school, among other areas. The therapist must ensure that the seating system fits in these environments. Factors such as accessibility into buildings, door widths, hall widths, table heights, sink heights, counter heights, and availability of accessible transportation need to be explored. The therapist should question the family about size, layout, and measurements of doorways in the home to ensure that the client can access all critical areas. The type of transportation the family uses should be noted. Whenever possible, the therapist should view and measure the family's van or car. If an electric wheelchair lift is used in a van, size and style of the lift are noted. Wheelchairs are held down in buses or vans by special locking systems mounted to the floor, known as wheelchair tie-downs. The location and type of the wheelchair tie-down is noted to ensure that it will accommodate the new wheelchair and seating. The family or teachers need to be questioned about school transportation and the school environment. The therapist should obtain information such as where the client's work area will be at work or school and whether the client will be able to access all necessary areas at work or school (bathrooms, cafeterias, classroom areas). Attention to the details of the client's environments and transportation systems ensures that the client will be able to access these areas and experience as much independence and autonomy as possible.

Compatibility With Other Technology

Often the client who is severely physically disabled requires a number of different types of technology to replace or augment functional or ADL skills. Some of those pieces of technology must be with the client at all times for the client to be truly independent. An example of this would be an augmentative communication device for a client who is nonverbal. This device needs to be safely mounted to the wheelchair on a sturdy mounting system where it is readily accessible. Incorporating the mounting of this or other devices used by the client into the original seating system is more cost-effective than trying to incorporate it after the fact. The therapist and seating team must be clear about all technology equipment goals during the seating evaluation to ensure that they are included in the design.

Initial Goals

After the evaluation data are collected and the hands-on evaluation is performed, the therapist begins to formulate and "build" postural goals. The initial goals are expressed by the section of the body being addressed, as shown in Table 2–1.

Table 2–1. FORMAT FOR INITIAL GOALS

Area	Problem	Goal
Pelvis		
Lower extremity		
Trunk		
Upper extremity		
Head		

The format of initial goals is explained in the following pages.

The Pelvis

As mentioned previously in the chapter, positioning goals begin at the pelvis and proceed to the lower extremities. This provides the client with a stable base of support. The seating surface should be firm enough to allow the ischial tuberosities to be level. A surface that is too soft or giving encourages asymmetrical postures. The ASISs should face forward. To ensure that the pelvis stays in the middle of the seat, it is supported on both lateral aspects. The posterior aspect of the pelvis, in the sacral area, is supported to encourage a neutral pelvic tilt. Pelvic deformities, such as a fixed posterior tilt or lateral obliquity must be accommodated. The goal in these cases should be to allow a forward-facing trunk and head, with the head in a balanced position. Failure to accommodate the deformities could result in the client sitting in poor compensatory postures to obtain sufficient stability to perform functional skills.

The Lower Extremities

The hips, knees, and feet are commonly positioned at 90-degree angles. This position provides the client with stability through the pelvis, thighs, and feet. Often this allows the client trunk and upper extremity mobility. An angle of *greater* than 90 degrees at the hips and knees may be necessary to break up or decrease extensor tone. Hips should be positioned at neutral rotation and abduction, although a larger degree of hip abduction may be needed to assist in breaking up extensor tone. Care must be taken to put seating supports that abduct the lower extremities distally and avoid the muscle belly area of the abductors along the medial thigh. Placement along the medial thigh can stimulate the abductors. Deformities at the hips, especially hip dislocation with adduction, are common, especially among clients with cerebral palsy and spina bifida. These deformities must be assessed carefully. In addition, attempting to move the lower extremities into a neutral position when there are hip contractures or restrictions will actually rotate the pelvis because the hips lack mobility. In this case, the deformities of the hips are accommodated with the goal of allowing the pelvis and trunk to face forward. Moving distally to the knees, knee angle is almost always dictated by flexibility, or lack of flexibility, of the hamstrings. The hamstrings cross the knees and hips and attach to the posterior pelvis to flex the knees and extend the hips. When hamstrings are even slightly tight, movement of the knee away from 90 degrees toward extension will posteriorly tilt the pelvis as the tight muscles stretch. Clients with very tight hamstrings may even have to have their knees positioned at greater than 90 degrees to decrease the pull on the posterior pelvis and maintain the pelvis in a neutral position. Failure to accommodate tight hamstrings results in the client sitting with a posteriorly rotated pelvis and a rounded trunk. In this position, the client will often appear to be constantly sliding down in the chair.

The feet are supported so that the ankle is flexed to 90 degrees, with even pressure between the heel and the ball of the foot. This prevents facilitation of the positive supporting reaction. Adding a strap over the ankle and positioning the foot to about 45 degrees of ankle dorsiflexion can further assist in decreasing pressure over the ball of the foot. Occasionally, clients may have developed plantar flexion contractures or other contractures of the ankle and foot. To protect the integrity of the hip and knee angles and to provide as much stability through the feet, these postures might be accommodated on the footrest.

The Trunk

With the base of support established, support of the trunk is addressed. Beginning proximally, the posterior pelvis is already well supported. It is often tempting to provide young children with lumbar supports to encourage low lumbar curvature and a slightly anteriorly tilted pelvis. This may be appropriate with teenagers and adults, but young children do not develop lumbar lordosis until between 8 and 12 years, so use of lumbar pads is inappropriate before this age (Zacharkow, 1988). Even in children 8 years of age or older, always remember to check movement at the knees when attempting to move the pelvis into even a slight anterior tilt because of the hamstrings' two-joint effect. Support of the trunk can extend to just below the inferior angle of the scapula if trunk control is good, or up to the level of the shoulders if control of the trunk is fair or poor. If the client has developed a fixed kyphosis or scoliosis, the counter and shape of the back must be accommodated. Otherwise, the client may touch the back component of the seating support system only at pressure points. In addition, failure to accommodate fixed trunk deformities may encourage further deformity.

Lateral trunk supports provide the client with some central stability to permit the development of distal (upper extremity) function. If the client has developed scoliosis, lateral supports can provide some corrective forces. However, a seating system does not *correct* deformities of the spine once they have occurred. It may slow the progression or lessen the extent of deformity, although this has not been supported through research. The only way to correct a deformity of the spine is through surgery, and the best means of supporting a spine with deformity is through the use of a body jacket. A body jacket (commonly known as a thoraco-lumbar-sacral orthosis) provides circumferential support, which a seating system that contacts the trunk only posteriorly and laterally cannot accomplish. Some individuals use body jackets once a deformity has developed. However, many individuals, for various reasons, are unable to tolerate a body jacket. In these cases, the corrective forces applied by a seating system are placed under the convex of the spinal curve and high on the opposite side. (*Note:* This therapy requires that the pelvis is well stabilized in midline. Lateral trunk supports used to provide these corrective forces without stabilizing the pelvis will result in the pelvis sliding laterally, rendering the lateral trunk supports ineffective.)

When the client has fair to poor trunk control, anterior trunk support is necessary to provide the client with additional central stability. The type and shape of the anterior supports vary. The goals are to provide just enough anterior trunk or shoulder support to guide the upper trunk into an upright position and allow functional activities to be performed by the upper extremities or to keep the head and shoulders in an upright, balanced position. Some clients require only anterior trunk support in the form of a horizontal chest strap to guide them into an upright position. Others require more aggressive anterior chest and shoulder support to inhibit the shoulders and upper back from falling or pulling into a kyphotic position. These supports are easily removable, so the therapist can work with the client to improve trunk control while the client is in the seating system. In addition, the caregiver can easily place the client into and out of the seating. However, the supports should not be removed outside of a therapy situation to make the client work on sitting up. It is unfair and inappropriate to expect a client to work on stabilizing himself or herself while expecting functional and ADL skills to be performed. Clients simply cannot do both at the same time.

Upper Extremities

Upper extremity support revolves around two goals: the physical or therapeutic goal of providing support to decrease the effects of tone or reflexes and the functional or ADL goal of providing an anterior work surface on which the upper extremities can perform these skills while the client is maintained in an appropriate position.

If the client has one or both functional upper extremities, the upper extremities need to be positioned so that they can move functionally. This will vary, depending on the client's neuromotor and orthopedic status. If the upper extremities are not functional, then they need to be supported in a position that accommodates any tonal or orthopedic problems or a position that is comfortable for the client. Usually upper extremity support is achieved through the use of a tray surface mounted on top of the wheelchair armrests or by replacing the armrests with arm supports. Many different supports are available, and the choice depends on the needs of the child. For example, blocks can be mounted behind the elbow area to discourage the abducted, externally rotated and retracted posture commonly seen in clients with cerebral palsy or traumatic brain injury. Some clients use a dowel or other grip on the tray to assist with stabilization so that the other arm can be used for function. Tray adaptations should not be a primary means of trunk control or support, especially with clients who must use one or both hands for function. The therapist should always look proximally first before adding distal support.

The Head

There are two main reasons to support the head: safety of clients being transported by bus or van in their chairs and therapeutic positioning. Every client who is transported while sitting in his or her wheelchair should have some type of headrest to provide posterior head protection similar to that available to a client riding in a car seat. This support should be removed if it is not needed at other times during the day.

Therapeutically, head supports are used when the client does not have sufficient control to balance his or her head and simultaneously attend to functional activities, for a client who requires something on which to "stabilize" his or her head to perform activities (such as a client with athetoid cerebral palsy), or for a client who displays a predominance of reflex activity (e.g., ATNR) that is elicited by head movement. When severe extensor tone or reflexes elicited by head movement are present, the head movements can be quite strong. In these cases, the headrest should be attached with sturdy hardware. Optimal or neutral head position may be unattainable for some clients due to the strength of the reflex. In these situations, the therapist may opt for the best compromise and allow a certain amount of abnormal positioning. Another group of clients are capable of "coming back" to a more neutral, midline position after going into an abnormal reflex or tonal posture. A more flexible or "dynamic" head positioning solution is appropriate for these individuals. Still other clients pull into a total flexion posture or are extremely hypotonic and are constantly sitting with their heads hanging down and their chins almost on their chests. This position leads to overstretched neck extensors, so that when these clients lift their heads up, they have a "gooseneck" posture of their head and neck. With these clients, an early introduction to a forehead band attached to a head support or even circumferential neck and head support may be necessary if the client is going to be in an upright position. These types of supports must be carefully evaluated to ensure that the client's oral-motor functions (especially swallowing) and breathing are not compromised. These types of anterior supports should never be used when the client is being transported in the chair, because serious neck injury could result in the event of an accident. However, a posterior head support should be included if the client is transported while sitting in the wheelchair, for the same reasons that we have headrests in our cars.

Simulation or Use of Trial Equipment

Once the therapist has determined initial goals through data collection and a thorough hands-on evaluation, those positioning goals must be tested. See Table 2–2 for an example of a full initial goal.

Table 2–2. INITIAL GOAL EXAMPLE

Area	Problem	Goal
Pelvis	Fixed obliquity to left; slides to left; bony ischial tuberosities	Accommodate pelvic obliquity to left; provide midline stability to decrease sliding to left; provide pressure-relieving surface under ischial tuberosities

This testing is done through a process called *simulation*. Simulation occurs in a device, usually a wheelchair base, in which various seating supports can be mounted and adjusted for individuals. Several seating manufacturers make multiadjustable devices on which many types of seating supports can be mounted. While these are useful for evaluation, they are also expensive, and not every team will have access to one. Another more readily available solution is to have several manual and powered wheelchairs into which an array of seating supports can be mounted and adjusted. Manufacturers and rehabilitation technology suppliers should be able to supply pieces of equipment on a short-term or long-term trial basis to a seating clinic (Fig. 2–5).

Simulation allows the therapist to test the viability of positioning goals with static pieces of equipment (Cook & Hussey, 1995). No matter how hard a therapist may try holding an individual with his or her hands, there is always some movement. In addition, there are not usually enough pairs of hands at the seating evaluation to fully support the client. Another crucial aspect of simulation is the opportunity to assess the functional and ADL skills while the client is in a simulated position to ensure that the client will be able to maintain or increase the level of function. For example, a client could be evaluated for his or her ability to use a powered wheelchair if the seating simulator were placed in a powered wheelchair base. Finally, simulation helps the therapist and the rehabilitation technology supplier, who will be ordering, fabricating, or assembling the equipment, to understand how the equipment is to function for each client. Measurements of the client are taken while the child is in the simulated position. (Please refer to the measurement section of the evaluation form, Appendix B.) The most accurate measurements of the client will be taken when he or she is in the optimal, simulated position.

Matching Final Goals to Equipment

At the conclusion of the simulation session, the therapist reviews initial goals, making any necessary changes for compilation of final goals. Although many times the final goals will be the same as initial goals, issues may have

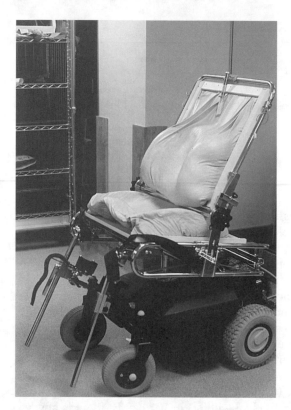

Figure 2–5. A multiadjustable seating simulator from Pin Dot Products mounted on an Invacare Arrow XT powered wheelchair base.

arisen during simulation that make initial goals unrealistic. For example, the client may have been unable to tolerate a certain position or the most desirable location of a support. Thus, the goals reflect a compromise between initial planning and information gained during the simulation session (Cook & Hussey, 1995).

As described previously, the therapist and other team members use a complex problem-solving process to arrive at equipment choices to meet identified goals. There are numerous pieces and types of seating supports and attachment hardware from many manufacturers. The primary responsibility for this part of the evaluation falls on the supplier as the equipment expert. The therapist and team must be clear about positioning goals so that these can be related to the supplier as accurately as possible. The positioning goals have to be matched with desired characteristics and location of support before a final equipment decision is made. Suppliers and the assessment team will need to consider characteristics of support, which include growth adjustability, flexibility, and type of materials necessary (e.g., firm foam, soft foam, waterproof or breathable fabrics). Different types of seating from various manufacturers can be combined to provide the most appropriate seating system for the client.

Table 2–3 is an example of a helpful system when matching goals to equipment. Location refers obviously to the part of the body that needs to be supported but also how much body contact is necessary to achieve control of the client's posture. If a client simply requires contact from seating support to encourage a midline or close to midline posture, then *planar* or *precontoured* seating supports will most likely be appropriate. These types of support can be taken off the shelf and put together in the most effective way for the individual client. Clients who require a lot of body contact because of severe tone or orthopedic deformities need a more customized approach, called *contoured* seating (Cook & Hussey, 1995).

Table 2–3. MATCHING GOALS TO EQUIPMENT

Area	Goal	Location and Characteristics	Solution
Pelvis	Encourage neutral, midline pelvis for 5-year-old boy with bony greater trochanters	Lateral pelvic support Adjustable in width for growth Well cushioned Waterproof covering	Adaptive engineering lateral pelvic supports, 1½ inches wide with 1 inch of foam-covered vinyl, mounted on 2-inch offset hardware to allow growth in width

THE FUNDING PROCESS

Seating equipment for children and adults is usually funded by private insurance, Medicaid (state funding), Medicare (federal funding for the elderly and those on disability), Children's Medical Services (called Crippled Children's Services in some states), or vocational rehabilitation. The most important thing a therapist has to investigate with each of these funding agencies is what type of equipment is paid for by each agency and what the funding limits are. The team must provide

- An itemized prescription (signed by the physician)
- A letter of medical necessity (signed by the physician)
- A copy of the team's evaluation

The funding agency may have additional requirements, depending on the insurance company or state in which the child resides.

The funding process usually follows this sequence:

1. Seating team provides the rehabilitation technology supplier with a prescription, evaluation note, and letter of medical necessity. The let-

ter of medical necessity provides an explanation of why each piece of equipment is needed. The letter of medical necessity should include the following information:

- The child's age, diagnosis, and prognosis
- A summary of evaluation findings (written less technically so the funding agency can understand)
- An explanation of why each piece of equipment is needed
- An estimate of how long it may last (to let them know growth and change is considered)

It is important to stress that this equipment is medically necessary. Pictures of the client before and after simulation are often included to help the funding agencies understand why the equipment is needed.

2. The rehabilitation technology supplier compiles a quote, which is an itemized list of the cost of each item. This is sent to the funding agency with all of the paperwork for approval (confirmation from the agency that funding is available before ordering the equipment).

3. Once prior approval is received, the rehabilitation technology supplier orders the equipment. When the equipment is received, the supplier assembles the equipment, and fits it to the individual in the seating clinic.

FITTING THE SEATING SYSTEM

If the seating system is carefully recommended, the fitting process will be straightforward. Adjustment of supports (such as lateral pelvic and thoracic supports), lap belts, and chest harnesses must be carried out with the individual in the seating system to ensure an appropriate fit.

Once the client has been fitted with the seating system, the therapist educates the client or caregiver on use and care of the system. Instruction on use includes how to build up the client's tolerance to the seating system, the activities for which the system is useful (if it is not being used all day), how to put the client properly in the seating system, and how to adjust belts and supports. Education cannot be stressed enough. The client, caregiver, and family who thoroughly understand how to use the seating system will ensure that it is successful.

CONCLUSION

If the therapist carefully gathers information from the team, client, and family; performs a thorough hands-on evaluation; and proceeds through simulation, the seating evaluation will be successful. Goals are matched to equipment in a systematic way to encourage the therapist, supplier, and other team members to find the best possible solutions for the client's needs.

STUDY QUESTIONS

1. Why is it important to consider the influence of primitive reflexes during a seating evaluation? Which reflexes must you evaluate?
2. What physical characteristics of a client may make it difficult or impossible to achieve "textbook" positioning in a wheelchair? What environmental characteristics may influence your ability to optimally position a client?

REFERENCES

Bergen, A., Presperin, J. & Tallman, T. (1990). *Positioning for function: Wheelchairs and other assistive technologies.* Valhalla, NY: Valhalla Rehab. Publications.

Colangelo, C. A. (1993). Biomechanical frame of reference. In P. Kramer & J. Hinojosa (Eds.), *Frames of reference for pediatric occupational therapy.* Baltimore: Williams and Wilkins.

Cook, A., & Hussey, S. (1995). *Assistive technologies: Principles and practice.* St. Louis, MO: Mosby–Yearbook.

Taylor, S. J. (1993). Wheelchair seating: A clinical framework for evaluation. *Occupational Therapy Practice, 4*(3), 51–58.

Taylor, S. J. & Trefler, E. (1984). Decision-making guidelines for seating and positioning children with cerebral palsy. In E. Trefler (Ed.), *Seating for children with cerebral palsy—A resource manual.* Memphis, University of Tennessee Rehabilitation Engineering Program.

Zacharkow, D. (1988). *Posture, sitting, standing, chair design and exercise.* Springfield, IL: Charles C Thomas.

BIBLIOGRAPHY

Bay, J. L. (1991). Positioning for head control to access an augmentative communication machine. *American Journal of Occupational Therapy 45,* 544–549.

Brubaker, C. E. (1986). Wheelchair prescription: An analysis of factors that affect mobility and performance. *Journal of Rehabilitation & Research Development, 23,* 19–26.

Cook, A., & Hussey, S. (1995). *Assistive technologies: Principles and practice.* St. Louis, MO: Mosby–Yearbook.

Fife, S. E., Roxborough, L. A., Armstrong, R. W., Harris, S. R., Gregson, J. L., & Field, D. (1991). Development of a clinical measure of postural control for assessment of adaptive seating in children with neuromotor disorders. Physical Therapy, *71,* 981–993.

Garber, S. L., Krouskop, T. A., & Carter, R. E. (1978). System for clinically evaluating wheelchair pressure relief cushions. *American Journal of Occupational Therapy, 32,* 565–570.

Hughes, C. J., Weimer, W. H., Sheth, P. N. & Brubaker, C. E. (1992). Biomechanics of wheelchair propulsion as a function of seat position and user-to-chair interface. *Archives of Physical Medicine and Rehabilitation, 73,* 263–269.

Hulme, J. B., et al. (1987). Behavior and postural changes observed with the use of adaptive seating by clients with multiple handicaps. Physical Therapy, *67,* 1060–1067.

Hulme, J. B., et al. (1987). Effects of adaptive seating devices on the eating and drinking of children with multiple handicaps. *American Journal of Occupational Therapy, 41,* 81–89.

Hulme, J. B., Bain, B., Hardin, M., McKinnon, A., & Waldron, D. (1989). The influence of adaptive seating devices on vocalization. *Journal of Communication Disorders, 22,* 137–145.

Luebben, A. (1992). Retrofitting: A case for community clinician input. Toronto, Ontario: Proceedings of the RESNA International Conference.

Luebben, A. (1989). Retrofitting: An unnecessary expense. Toronto, Ontario: Proceedings of the RESNA International Conference.

Medhat, M. A., & Hobson, D. A. (1992). *Standardization of terminology and descriptive methods for specialized seating.* Washington, DC: RESNA Press.

McCormack, D. J. (1990). The effects of keyguard use and pelvic positioning on typing speed and accuracy in a boy with cerebral palsy. *American Journal of Occupational Therapy, 44,* 312–315.

Nwaobi, O. M. (1987). Non-dominant arm restraint and dominant arm function in a child with athetoid cerebral palsy: EMG and functional evaluation. *Archives of Physical Medicine and Rehabilitation, 68,* 837–839.

Nwaobi, O. M., & Smith, P. D. (1986). Effect of adaptive seating on pulmonary function in children with cerebral palsy. *Developmental Medicine and Child Neurology, 28,* 351–354.

Rodgers, M. N., Gayle, G. W., Figoni, S. E., Kobayashi, M., Glaser, R. M., & Gupta, S. C. (1992). Kinematic and kinetic responses to wheelchair propulsion during fatigue in spinal cord injured individuals—A pilot study. Toronto, Ontario: Proceedings of the RESNA International Conference.

Steel, K. O., Glover, J. E., & Spasoff, R. A. (1991). The motor control assessment: An instrument to measure motor control in physically disabled children. *Archives of Physical Medicine and Rehabilitation, 72,* 549–553.

Zacharkow, D. (1988). *Posture, sitting, standing, chair design and exercise.* Springfield, IL: Charles C Thomas.

A Clinical Framework for the Evaluation for Wheelchair Seating and Mobility

Primary staff

Therapist or rehabilitation technology supplier is present to listen.

Therapist and rehabilitation technology supplier

Therapist or rehabilitation technology supplier sometimes assists at the direction of the therapist if extra "hands" needed.

1. Information-gathering and needs assessment

- Client goals
- Medical and surgical histories, including planned procedures that would affect seating or mobility, (e.g., orthopedic surgery)
- Current and desired functional and activities of daily living (ADL) skills, including other types of technology that need to be integrated into the seating or mobility unit (e.g., an augmentative communication device)
- Discussion of available funding sources
- Environmental considerations, including home accessibility, transportation used, and review of current equipment, including measurements (current and potential future environments)
- Site visit if it is determined that more accessibility information is necessary
- Coordinate with other professionals (e.g., therapists, physicians, rehabilitation engineers)

2. Physical evaluation and hands-on mat evaluation

- Orthopedic status, including joint mobility, which joints are *fixed* contractures, which are *flexible*. Therapist begins to feel how much and what type of support or accommodation will be necessary to place that client in a functional seated posture.
- Neuromotor status. Therapist feels and observes the effects of abnormal tone and reflexes on the client's posture, including what positions and movement initiate this tone.
- Sensory status, including skin inspection and history of pressure sores

3. Synthesis of evaluation findings and development of initial postural goals

Therapist and client

- Goals are expressed using anatomic areas as follows:
  - □ Pelvis
  - □ Lower extremities
  - □ Trunk
  - □ Upper extremities
  - □ Head
  - □ Mobility, ADL, functional skills
- This forces the therapist to synthesize evaluation findings and think through goals, beginning with the base of the client's support, at the pelvis.
- These are initial goals only and must actually be tested before being finalized.

4. Simulation

Therapist and rehabilitation technology supplier

- This phase allows testing of initial goals with static pieces of equipment. This can occur in a seating simulator produced by one of several manufacturers or in a manual or powered wheelchair base with various types of seat, back, and other components. Rehabilitation technology supplier often provides equipment for simulation, either from his or her own stock or through arrangement with a manufacturer.
- Therapist and rehabilitation technology supplier are now beginning to match therapeutic goals to equipment characteristics.
- Functional and ADL skills (e.g., mobility, feeding) can be tested in the simulated position to determine if initial goals facilitate or inhibit replication of these skills.
- When powered and manual wheelchairs are being tested, the client is given the opportunity to push or drive the chair, take the chair apart for transportation, and fit it in the car, truck, or van.
- Goals are finalized at this time as the client provides feedback and the therapist observes the effects of the maintained position. They are finalized in the same format as the initial goals.
- Measurements are taken while the client is in a simulated position because this is the position in which he or she will be sitting.

5. Order specification: Matching final goals to equipment

Rehabilitation technology supplier and therapist

- Therapist provides information on needed characteristics of equipment (e.g., pressure relieving, adjustable), while the rehabilitation technology supplier matches those characteristics to possible commercial or customized solutions.
- Rehabilitation technology supplier outlines funding needs for preferred equipment or product options that could match available funding.
- Rehabilitation technology supplier identifies specific product ordering information, ensuring that various components will work together in the seating and mobility unit.
- This is all done for funding justification and, after funding is approved, for ordering and assembly.

6. Funding, assembly or fabrication, delivery

Therapist

- Provides evaluation report and letter of justification (including photos when necessary) and coordinates obtaining prescription
- Sends information to rehabilitation technology supplier
- Participates in setup and fitting to ensure products meet client's goals
- Provides client with training on appropriate use of the equipment

Rehabilitation technology supplier

- Provides cost and evaluation information to funding source
- Tracks status of requests
- Assembles equipment and checks against original order
- Participates in fitting to ensure products are adjusted properly
- Educates client on product care and maintenance, warranty information, and repair information

Information Necessary for the Claims Process for Rehabilitative and Assistive Technology

The individual submitting the claim should obtain the necessary information from the clinical framework.

The packet of information includes the physician's prescription(s), evaluation report, and reviewer's worksheet.

Submitter's worksheet

The following client has undergone an evaluation for seating or mobility:

Name _____

Date of evaluation _____ Date of birth _____

Diagnosis _____

Related diagnoses _____

_____

_____

Medicare number _____

Was an occupational or physical therapist involved in any part of the evaluation?

Y/N

If so, name and telephone

number _____

The following checklist is to ensure this information is included in the evaluation.

A. **This request is for:**
1. A new wheelchair (write evaluation report)
2. New seating components (write evaluation report)
3. Repairs and supplies
   If yes, state age of components being replaced and reasons for replacement, if known.

B. **Needs assessment and information gathering**
1. Client goals
2. Medical and surgical histories
3. Current functional and activities of daily living (ADL) skills, including other types of assistive technology the client uses to achieve these skills
4. Cognitive status
5. Inventory and measurement of current seating or mobility equipment
6. Desired functional and ADL skills
7. Recommended equipment compatible with current environment?
8. Type of transportation available to client

C. **Physical evaluation**
1. List any range of motion limitations that would preclude client from obtaining a 90-90-90 seated posture; indicate whether fixed or flexible.
   a. Pelvis
   b. Lower extremities
   c. Trunk
   d. Upper extremities
   e. Head
   Surgical intervention planned for limitations?
   List any other relevant orthopedic conditions:

   _____

2. Indicate presence of abnormal tone and reflexes:
   a. Type of tone and severity
   b. Type of reflexes
   c. Impact of tone or reflexes on function

   _____

3. Gross motor function (once supported):
   trunk balance-
   head control-

   _____

4. Skin condition
   a. Sensation absent or impaired? Where?
   b. Method of relieving pressure
      Grade and location of any pressure sores
   c. Client at high risk for development of sores? If yes, why?

    d. Surgical intervention planned for sores?
    e. Has the client ever had surgery for pressure sores?

5. Was trial equipment (seating) used with the client to obtain desired positions and test functional and ADL skills?
    a. Include picture of the client before and after trial with equipment.
    b. Were the client's goals met? Were additional goals realized?

Intervention goals	*Solutions*
1. Pelvis	
2. Lower extremities	
3. Trunk	
4. Upper extremities	
5. Head	
6. Orientation in space	

6. For powered and manual mobility devices, before specific equipment is recommended, the following questions must be answered:
   a. Was recommended or similar mobility device tried in client's vehicle or residence?
   b. Does the client have only household ambulation?
   c. Is the client able to propel a manual wheelchair? If not, why?
   d. Where does the client primarily intend to use the device?
   e. Did client have the opportunity to propel or drive the device?

   For powered devices:
   a. How did the client drive it?
      — Standard joystick
      — Standard joystick with nonstandard position (special interfacing hardware)
      — Specialty control (e.g., single switches, sip and puff, head controller)
   b. If other than standard joystick used, list functional reasons special placement or control used:

   c. For standard joystick, functionally justify use of other than basic electronics:

   For manual devices:
   a. List features and why needed:

APPENDIX C

Resources

The American Occupational Therapy Association (AOTA) has a special interest section on technology. Call AOTA headquarters for more information.

The International Seating Symposium alternates yearly between Vancouver, British Columbia, and Pittsburgh, Pennsylvania (1996—Vancouver, 1997—Pittsburgh). In Canada, contact David Cooper or Lori Roxborough at (604)436-1743. For the Pennsylvania conference, contact Elaine Trefler at (412)647-1270.

RESNA—A society for the advancement of rehabilitative and assistive technologies. This organization has a special interest group called "Seating and Wheeled Mobility," composed of about 600 members. In addition, they have a yearly conference, a journal called "*Assistive Technology*," and bimonthly newsletter. For further information, please contact RESNA, 1700 N. Moore Street, Suite 1540, Arlington, VA, 22209-1903. The phone numbers are (703)524-6686, TTY/TDD; (703)524-6639.

TEAM Rehabilitation Report is a magazine focused on assistive technologies. Free subscription is available to professionals. For further information, please call (800)543-4116.

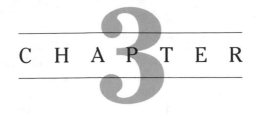

CHAPTER 3

ACCESS METHODS

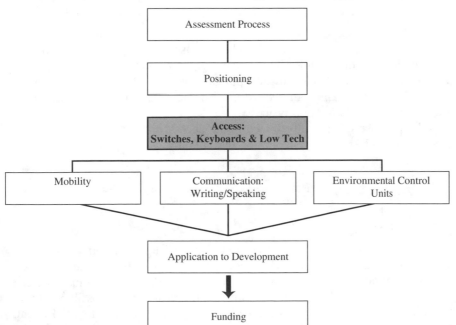

Assistive Technology Guide

Assessment Process

Positioning

**Access:
Switches, Keyboards & Low Tech**

Mobility

Communication:
Writing/Speaking

Environmental Control
Units

Application to Development

Funding

The access assessment takes place after preliminary seating and positioning issues have been addressed. At times, due to the distance the client must travel for the assessment, it is a one-time assessment; at other times, it is ongoing. Yorkston and Carlan (1986) recommend the ongoing approach to assessment, which is the method presented throughout this book. It is necessary to re-evaluate as the client's needs change, motor control develops, cognitive abilities increase, and available technology improves.

Access is the key to the rest of technology operation. Access is defined as the point of contact between the person and the assistive technology (AT). Access is the point at which the user comes into contact with the input device by using a limb, finger, or toe to press a switch or key. It is this point of connecting with the AT device that the word *access* describes. As indicated in the illustration on the previous page and as described in the Human-Environment/Technology Interface Model (Smith, 1991), access determines how the user will interface with the AT devices. Access therefore is a critical link between the user and the devices. Appropriate access leads the user to independence. Without appropriate access, the best assistive device cannot be adequately used by the individual. Access needs to be properly evaluated, or the doors to completing tasks with greater independence will be partially closed or shut because the individual will need more time to accomplish tasks or will not be able to do them at all. Here are two examples:

1. If the individual is using a standard keyboard but having difficulty reaching all the keys, efficiency may be impaired.
2. An individual with C3–4 quadriplegia who wants to drive a powered wheelchair will want access methods that do not require motor control of the hand.

When access methods are carefully chosen, users with physical disabilities can use devices more fully. This means greater independence in writing, speaking, driving a wheelchair, and pursuing academic and recreational activities. Therapists trained in access assessments make a major contribution to this part of the evaluation process.

The purpose of carefully selecting the access method(s) when using AT devices is to enhance five factors, the individual's:

1. Speed
2. Accuracy
3. Control
4. Reliability
5. Endurance

These five factors must be in the forefront of the therapist's mind as the access assessment progresses. Using AT devices can be a slow process that the user may find frustrating. When evaluating access methods, keep in mind the need to recommend methods that the individual can use as fast as possible without jeopardizing accuracy. Therefore, *speed,* making the system fast, yet efficient, is of utmost importance. The individual must also be able to control the AT devices accurately. Without *accuracy,* use of the AT device is impeded. Limited accuracy can lead to the device sitting on a shelf and not being used. *Control* can be likened to independence. Individuals with full control of their AT devices can fully operate them without assistance. *Reliability* refers to the consistency with which an individual must be able to complete a motor act to activate the AT device. Considering reliability in access leads to the proper keyboard or switch recommendation and placement. Some *endurance* is needed. The access method should not cause undue strain or create a state of tiredness. Keeping these five factors in mind during the assessment helps the therapist recommend appropriate access methods that will increase the individual's ability to use AT devices. These factors influence the effectiveness of the device, how frequently it is used, and the individual's independence.

ACCESS METHODS

Before describing the access assessment process, two terms need to be defined, direct selection and indirect selection. These two methods form the foundation for most input strategies. Therapists working in AT must understand the characteristics of these methods and the positive and negative attributes of each.

Direct Selection

Direct selection is an access method in which each item of the selection set is available at any time to the user. Using the computer keyboard to type the letters of the alphabet is an example of direct selection. Every symbol needed to spell any English word is equally available at any time. The user can press the "P" key just as easily as he or she can press the "A" key. Direct selection is usually faster than indirect selection.

Indirect Selection

Indirect selection is an access method in which more than one step is required in the selection process (i.e., it is indirect). For this method, one or more switches are used for selection. For efficiency, switches are used with a technique called *scanning.* Scanning provides access to a selection set, such as the alphabet, icon, or pictures. When using scanning with one or more switches, only one item in the selection set is available at any time. For example, if the alphabet is the selection set, and the individual wants to spell his name, "David," he must press the switch to activate the cursor, wait for the cursor to pass over the "A, B, C," and be ready to press the switch again when the cursor highlights the "D." The process must be repeated for each remaining letter in the name. A difficulty associated with scanning is the timing of switch activation. If the switch is not pressed precisely when the cursor highlights the letter of choice, then an error occurs. The user must wait until the cursor passes over the item again. Referring to the example of David, if he anticipates the cursor movement and presses the switch too soon, the letter "C" appears on the display; if he waits too long, the letter "E" appears. The advantage of scanning is that reliable motor control is needed only over one movement. The disadvantage is that usually it is slower than direct selection and requires a higher cognitive capability. Additional information on scanning is in Appendix A.

PRELIMINARY ASSESSMENT INFORMATION

Before beginning the assessment, it is important to know the individual's degree of involvement with primitive reflexes. Primitive reflexes can hinder the individual's ability to access a switch or keyboard. Reflexes may need to be tested, or notes from the therapist who regularly treats this individual, which were sent in the pre-evaluation form, may contain this information. Questions to be answered include, "Is the individual sensitive to any primitive reflexes?" "How strong is the response?" "What triggers the reflex?" "Can proper seating help encourage appropriate posturing and discourage triggering a reflex?"

INTERACTIONS DURING THE ASSESSMENT

As the assessment progresses, the therapist must remember that the client will be using the access method(s). The client and the therapist or AT team are together solving a puzzle. They are asking the question, "Where is (are) the best access site(s) to be found?" The client should feel involved, and his or her choices need to be kept foremost in the mind of the therapist. If the client appears to have better head than hand control but feels that the head-access method makes him or her look foolish and prefers using his or her hand, then the client and therapist need to compromise on the access site. The final decision rests with the client. It may be that devices that need to be used frequently are accessed by one site, and devices that are used only once or twice a day are accessed by a different site.

ASSESSMENT

The therapist should first observe the client's motor control and current access method(s) (Fig. 3–1), including all systems the client currently uses, such as those for controlling a personal mobility device, computer access, communication access, pointing, gesturing, and eye gaze. While observing, it is important to keep in mind the five factors (see page 44) important to enhancing access.

The assessing therapist will then evaluate the individual to observe whether the current access method is truly the most appropriate. The therapist

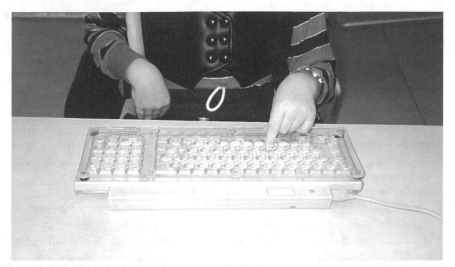

Figure 3–1. Individual using current access method.

may decide to try to improve the access method that the individual already uses by reviewing the individual's control using a variety of control sites and methods.

Direct selection using some part of the hand should be considered first (Goosens' & Crain, 1992). Direct selection is usually faster than scanning methods and is cognitively easier to understand. Hand access, using one or both hands or arms, is tried first because most objects are accessed this way by individuals without disabilities. The individual being assessed has observed other people using their hands to operate devices and manipulate objects, so using the hand provides a sense of normalcy to any activity (Campbell, 1985).

The therapist will find information from the treating therapist and family members valuable. These individuals have had the opportunity to work with the client longer and therefore usually know where the client's strengths lie. Comments like "She can control her head movement to the left but not the right" can help direct the assessment. At times, proper positioning will provide control that the client had not previously demonstrated. At other times, the client's strengths in movement will not be clear, and the team will work together to discover the body part(s) over which the client has more control. Although the assessing therapist should not overlook new or different areas of potential control, relying on the information from people who know the client well can help guide the initial parts of the assessment.

There are several components to keep in mind when considering direct selection. These are the size of the items, the amount of space needed between the items, and the position and location. These factors are discussed one at a time. Assessments for indirect selection are then described.

Direct-Selection Components

Size of Individual Items

Two grids, each on an 18 × 12-inch piece of cardboard or tagboard, can be made for this part of the assessment. One board should be marked off as a grid of 1 × 1-inch squares, the other into 2 × 2-inch squares (Figs. 3–2 and 3–3). The squares can be numbered and laminated to protect them, so that stickers can be applied and removed multiple times without damaging the board. Color or animal stickers are used, depending on the individual's age, familiarity with these objects, and cognitive ability. To increase motivation, children can be asked to select the animal stickers they would like to use. At the end of each trial, the sticker can be placed on the child's shirt or back of the hand, and new stickers are chosen for each new trial. After stickers are placed on various squares on the board, the individual is asked to point to the various squares where the stickers have been placed. If the individual has trouble pointing accurately using the 1 × 1-inch squares, then the board with the 2 × 2-inch squares should be tried to determine whether larger targets increase accuracy. If 1 × 1-inch squares pose no difficulty, then keyboard access should be examined. Once the individual's accuracy is determined to be in the range of the 2 × 2-inch squares, 1 × 1-inch squares, or

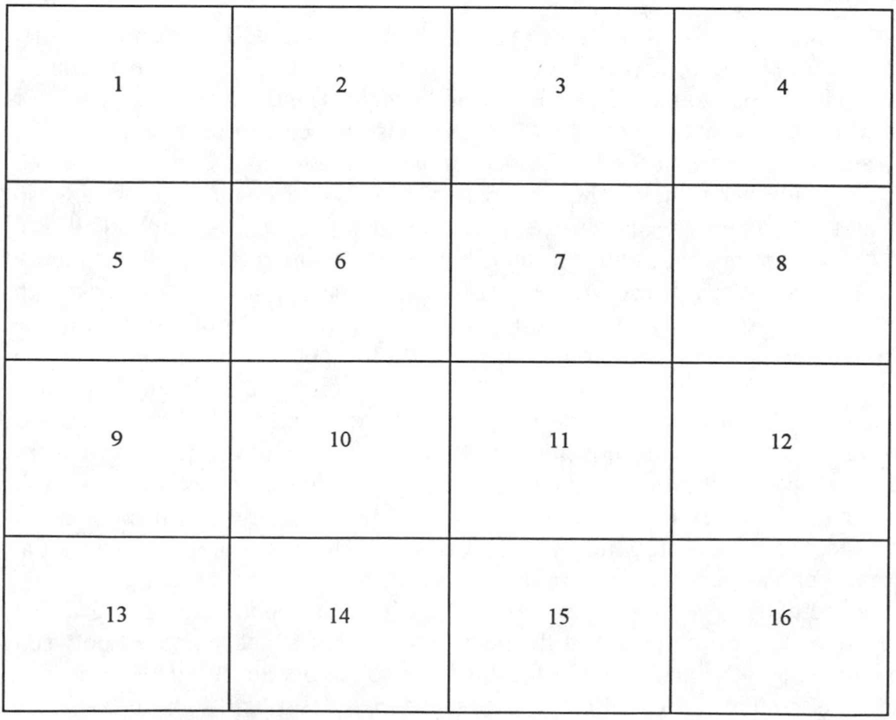

1	2	3	4
5	6	7	8
9	10	11	12
13	14	15	16

Figure 3–2. 2 × 2-inch grid.

1	2	3	4	5	6
7	8	9	10	11	12
13	14	15	16	17	18
19	20	21	22	23	24
25	26	27	30	31	32
33	34	35	36	37	38

Figure 3–3. 1 × 1-inch grid.

a standard "qwerty" keyboard (the standard keyboard letter arrangement used on all computer keyboards), the therapist can review the available keyboards with the appropriate key size to meet the individual's goals.

Amount of Space Needed Between Items

At times, it appears that the items are the appropriate size for the individual to indicate his or her choice, but additional blank space is needed between items so the individual can clearly indicate his or her selection to others. In this situation, the assessment begins with stickers placed on adjacent squares. The individual is asked to point to the various stickers on the board. The stickers are moved farther apart until the individual can clearly delineate to which sticker he or she is pointing (Fig. 3–4).

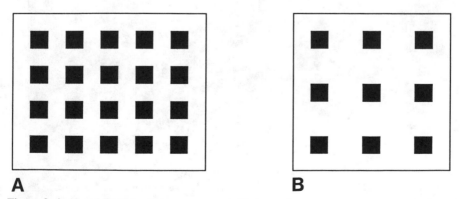

A   **B**

Figure 3–4. (*A* and *B*) Determining space needed between items.

Position and Location of the Board

The tag board should be placed on the individual's lap tray, which should have been properly fitted during the seating and positioning assessment. Optimally, the tray allows 90-degree elbow flexion and does not promote shoulder elevation or slouching. Testing usually begins by placing either the 1 × 1-inch or the 2 × 2-inch grid tag board at the individual's midline. The board can be moved to the right or left or placed at an angle, depending on where the individual appears to have greatest control over his or her movements. Some individuals prefer to stay on the same side of the midline and not cross it; others show a greater ability to cross the midline as they stabilize their forearms against their trunks or lap trays. In the latter situation, the tag board is usually placed more at an angle.

At times, inclining the board gives the individual the additional assistance needed to achieve accuracy when pointing to the stickers on the board. Some individuals will demonstrate more control if they are able to rest their forearm on the tag board, which is slightly elevated. This provides more control for pointing. Incline surfaces can be fabricated with wood. Three-ring binders can be used for assessment purposes and are discussed in Chapter 5 (Fig. 3–5).

In the assessment of direct selection access, tag boards can be used with handheld pointers, head pointers, or a toe. This all depends on the individual's capabilities. The Green Dot Test (discussed later in this chapter) can be used with the types of grids just described to provide quantitative information. If after exhausting all possibilities for direct selection, the individual is unable to reliably and consistently control either the hand with handheld devices, the head using a head pointer, or the toe, then indirect selection using switches should be considered.

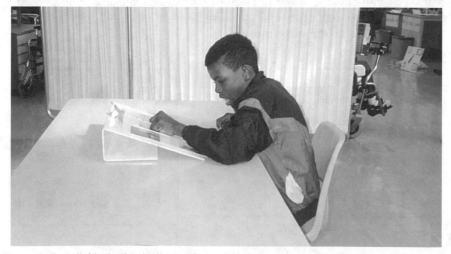

Figure 3–5. Individual using incline surface to improve access.

Mice and Track Balls

Mice and track balls are standard input devices needed to run many software packages. Many different mice and track balls are available. Some mice are scaled down in size to fit the smaller hands of children. A track ball is an upside-down mouse. The ball sits in a base and is typically moved with the fingers. As the ball is moved, the cursor responds on the screen. Track balls may be easier to use for people who have limited motor control. Several mice and track balls should be made available so individuals can get the feel of how each responds.

Features to consider when evaluating mice and track balls are the location and size of the buttons, which make them easy or difficult to reach and press, and the amount of pressure needed to activate the buttons. In addition, the size and drag of the ball should be evaluated when investigating track balls. Some individuals find double clicking difficult. Some mice now have buttons specifically programmed to double click when pressed once.

If the individual has some control over the mouse but motor control is considered poor, the therapist needs to analyze the task involved and assess where the difficulties lie. A test can be developed using each mouse or track ball. This can be done with a drawing or word processor program. The necessary tasks the client needs to be able to perform are dragging, clicking, and moving objects around the screen. For each mouse or track ball, the individual should go through the series of movements, such as opening a computer file, drawing a box, and filling the box in with a color. Another team member should time how long it takes the individual to complete all the tasks, take notes on ease of use and change in muscle tone, and provide anecdotal comments. This assessment provides the team with qualitative and quantitative information on each mouse and track ball that can be used when making recommendations.

Currently, most software programs are designed so that all the mouse commands have keyboard equivalents. Further, operating systems for both the Macintosh and PCs have "mouse keys." Mouse keys allow the number pad to be used to direct the cursor as if the user were moving the mouse. For Macintosh computers, this feature, called Easy Keys, comes with the computer. For PCs, Access Pack for Microsoft Windows, distributed by Microsoft, eliminates the problem of using the mouse.

Indirect-Selection Components

Once again, the hand or arm, head or foot, or knee may be considered potential access sites. For the same reasons discussed in the previous section on direct selection, using the hand to activate a switch is usually evaluated first. The tag boards can again be used to investigate switch placement on the lap tray. The switch is usually placed in the midline first and then moved from one side to the other, depending on the individual's motor skill to press the switch on command. At times, placing the switch on an incline to slant it or recessed within a lap tray improves the individual's ability to accurately press it.

When considering head control, the type of head movement must be addressed so that primitive reflexes are not triggered. Generally, a lateral tilt of the head is preferred to any other movement (Goosens' & Crain, 1992). Neck flexion can cause the asymmetrical tonic neck reflex; extension can cause hyperextension. Turning the head to the left or right can cause the asymmetrical tonic neck reflex. For people with abnormal nervous system function, these neck movements can cause unwanted tone in the body. A lateral head tilt usually does not elicit undesirable reflexes and does not require a large arc of excursion (Fig. 3–6). This is not a natural movement and thus must be taught. In addition, when using this head movement, the individual may not be able to see the switch. Training time must be provided during the assessment and afterwards so that the individual can become accustomed to the switch placement. Once optimal switch placement has been decided, it is critical to maintain the switch in that position so that the individual can practice finding and pressing the switch using his or her head.

The foot or knee can also be assessed for switch access. As with the head, when the foot or knee is used, the switch may not be in the line of vision. The assessing therapist needs to allow time for the individual to become accustomed to the movement pattern he or she is being asked to perform. Pressing a switch with the knee or foot is not a natural movement, and the individual will need time to learn what he or she is supposed to do. For the knee, the movement can be a slight increase of hip flexion, abduction, or adduction. Typically, the foot movement assessed is internal or external rotation when the foot is positioned in neutral. When using this placement for a switch, the therapist must ensure that it does not interfere with transfers.

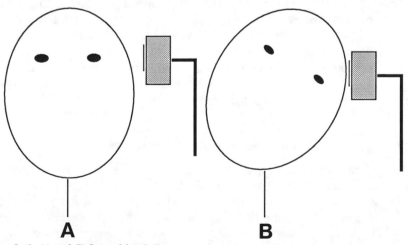

Figure 3–6. (*A* and *B*) Lateral head tilt.

Single-Switch Components

Types of switches and assessment of switches are described in Chapter 4. The switch should first be placed at the site(s) where the therapist and family suspect that the individual has the most control. It should then be connected to an age-appropriate toy or computer with a game or other interesting software. Place the switch at these sites one at a time. The activity should be appropriate for the age and cognitive level of the individual being tested. If the individual is a child, the child can be asked to make the toy move: "We want to see the bear dance; if you press this switch with your foot, the bear will dance for us. Press the switch!" If the individual is an adult, the process of finding an appropriate switch placement is explained, and the adult presses the switch to the best of his or her ability. Once the individual has the basic idea of switch pressing, the next level is to ask the individual to perform this act only when asked to do so. Phrases can be used such as "Only press the switch when I say 'go.' 1, 2, 3, Go." This helps the therapist assess the individual's ability to press the switch on command. This factor is important when using scanning—pressing the switch only when it is over the desired selection, not before and not after.

In addition, the individual must be able to release the switch on command. This relates to the ability to release the switch in a scanning array to indicate the desired item. The individual can be told, "Now, I want you to hold the switch down and don't let go until I tell you to. OK, press your switch; keep holding it down! OK, let go."

The next motor control to assess is the ability to press the switch in a sequence—for instance, pressing the switch three times sequentially and then releasing it. This helps to indicate if the individual has enough control to use row and column scanning. Phrases can be used such as "I will hold up my fingers, and I want you to press your switch as many times as the number of fingers I show you." The number of fingers should change for each trial. Keeping score on the number of times the individual was able to perform this activity for each switch site used can help in the recommendation phase of switch and body location.

The ability to adequately control a switch may not happen in one session. Single-switch access may be the access method of choice if the individual can press the switch on command. The other attributes needed for switch use may come later with training.

Eye Pointing

Although eye pointing is a direct-selection method, it appears last in this section because it is generally the access method considered after all other potential methods have been exhausted. Usually, individuals have more control over their eyes than any other part of their body. The eyes have the closest connection to the brain. Therefore, if the individual cannot control other body parts reliably, he or she may be able to control the eyes (Blackstone, 1986). In many cases, eye pointing uses low-technology equipment. This means that the user will not be able to store messages for later retrieval or call someone when they wish to speak. The listener must always be present to receive the message and wait as the user spells out each letter of each word or directs the eyes to icons or pictures. Thus, this method is slow, which is another reason it is one of the last access methods to be considered.

To investigate the feasibility of using this method, the therapist should ask the individual to point to one of two pictures using the eyes. The therapist should hold up the pictures, one on the left and one on the right. More pictures are introduced to examine what size the pictures need to be and how far apart they need to be spaced so that a clear distinction can be made when the individual is eye pointing. The individual can also spell using this method. When spelling, an E-Tran board is used. Additional information on E-Tran can be found in Chapter 7.

Summary

Once an access site has been narrowed to one or two potentially useful sites, training can begin with the treating therapist. Many of the movements that the individual has been asked to perform are not natural, and it is perhaps the first time the individual has tried to purposefully move in this way. The treating therapist needs to be instructed as to how she or he can assist the individual in practicing these movements so that they become natural and can be used to press a switch to control a toy, a computer, or some element of the environment. Natural use of these movements will come only with practice. At the same time, the family, treating therapist, and AT therapist will be looking toward the future. Even if the individual does not use direct selection now, he or she may develop more motor control at a later time.

Questions for the Therapist

Therapists play an invaluable role in access assessments. In most cases, they will keep in mind the following questions as they begin to identify the individual's strengths in motor control:

- What is the smallest area to which the individual can accurately and dependably point?
- Does this indicate using a keyboard, or should the evaluation proceed to switch use?
- Can the individual accurately press a switch?
- Which body part, in what position, gives the individual optimal control over the switch?
- Can this skill be taught to the individual?
- Which type of switch provides the individual with the best feedback?
- Should two switches in different locations be considered?

- Over which switch does the individual have more control?
- What areas are readily available in the individual's visual field?
- What colors can the individual see the best?
- Are there visual-field cuts?

Answers to these questions provide information to help therapists strategically place items so that the individual has as much visual information as possible from the communication symbol set. This knowledge prevents placement of symbols or symbol sets in areas where the individual has limited vision. In addition, therapists should evaluate the size of items to ensure that they are large enough for the individual to see clearly. Symbols that are too small or intricately drawn may increase errors.

ASSESSMENT TOOLS
Direct Selection

The Green Dot Test

The Green Dot Test, developed at the Trace Center, is an excellent tool to quantify keyboard ability (Smith, 1992). To administer the test, place six stickers on six peripheral keys of the keyboard being tested. The peripheral keys are used to note the range of motion needed to operate each particular keyboard. The sticker that the individual presses first can be any one of the marked keys. The path the individual uses to press the keys and the starting position of the limb for the test should be consistent throughout each trial for each keyboard. The therapist may want to write down the key with which the individual begins, such as the "A" key or the "return" key, so that this key will be used with successive trials and keyboards. It is also important to keep the starting position consistent. Using the index finger as an example, the starting position can be the individual's finger hovering over the first key or the individual's arm resting on the lap tray. Either position is suitable but must be consistent throughout the testing process for all trials on all keyboards so that comparison between keyboards will have meaning.

The test is performed a minimum of three times. Three trials can be used to calculate the average speed with which the individual can press the keys on a particular keyboard. It is usually faster for the individual to use a smaller keyboard with keys that are closer together. However, the individual's accuracy and ability to press the individual keys without pressing adjacent keys must also be considered during the assessment (error rate). Other information that should be gathered by the therapist while the individual performs the test includes overall ease during key pressing, fatigue rate, and amount of effort involved. Did the individual appear to be working very hard, or were the movements smooth and graceful? What was the overall level of tension in the body?

The Green Dot Test is so named because green stickers were first used in the testing procedures. As discussed previously, colorful stickers with faces or pictures of animals, which may be more enticing to younger children, can be used in place of the green stickers. This test focuses on motor skills and, to the extent possible, eliminates the cognitive component of typing. The only special tools needed are stickers and a stopwatch or watch with a second hand. No special software is needed. The individual does not need to watch the screen while performing the test.

It is not necessary to have the keyboard connected to a computer for this test. However, additional information can be collected if the keyboard is used with a computer and a word processor is loaded into memory. With use of a word processor, the errors are displayed on the screen; this eliminates guessing or keeping count of error rate. Also, hand dragging over the keys can indicate the need for a keyguard or software that prevents keys from repeating when pressed for long periods of time. Finally, the computer can calculate multiple key presses. This information is displayed on the screen. It can then be printed out, tabulated, and compared with other keyboard results.

Keyboard Assessment Program

The Keyboard Assessment Program (KAP) was developed by the Assistive Device Center at California State University, Sacramento (Cook, 1988). Although this program runs on dated equipment, namely the Apple II family and GS computers, it is included here because these types of computers remain in use. This program tests three basic elements: the ability to

1. Press a single key when directed
2. Press a series of preselected keys when directed
3. Simultaneously press two keys when directed (i.e., press the control key and a letter key simultaneously)

Correct answers, errors, and speed are stored on a disk and can be printed out. This program, like the Green Dot Test, provides the clinician with quantitative information regarding the individual's ability to use the Apple IIe or GS keyboard.

For some individuals, using direct selection may be too difficult for their motor ability but should be reconsidered at a later time. Other assessment tools test individuals' ability to scan. These tools are used when direct selection appears to be too difficult.

Scanning Tests

Single-Input Control Assessment

The Single-Input Control Assessment software program (Don Johnston Incorporated) runs on the Apple II family and GS computers. It helps to quantify the user's skill using the head or limbs to activate a switch. The user needs to attend to the screen while preparing to press the switch.

This test has three components that relate to three aspects of single-switch use: (1) response task, (2) autoscan task, and (3) hold/release task. The purpose of the response task is to measure the time it takes to respond to a visual stimulus on the computer screen and press the switch and the length of time the switch is held down. This allows the therapist to obtain information on the type of switch being used, the length of time the switch was held down, and the number of prehits. This information can be valuable as the individual is observed using various switches and switch positions.

The autoscan task tests the user's ability to use an automatic linear scan. The scanning interval is fixed. The data collected during this task are target position, when the user presses the switch, number of times the cursor goes back to the beginning of the scan, response time when the switch is pressed, and holding time.

The hold/release task tests the individual's holding down the switch for a set length of time. This action is important because some access programs require that the individual hold the switch down and release it at a set time. Inverse scanning is an example of such a program. Data collected are number of attempts at holding for each trial, maximum hold time, and release time.

While evaluating the three aspects of single-switch use, the clinician can change the switch, switch position, and then compare scores. This provides quantifiable data to help in making decisions regarding switch options.

Scanning Assessment Tool

The Scanning Assessment Tool software program runs on a Macintosh computer (Angelo, 1992). It was designed to test the three scanning modes at the basic level. With this tool, the therapist determines the number of boxes (three, six, or nine) to be scanned, the speed the cursor moves across the boxes, and when the cursor begins to move. The program collects information on scanning mode, cursor speed, switches used, and switch position. The data are displayed in table or graph formats and can be printed out. To use a switch with this program, the Ke:nx or Macintosh Switch Interface, both available from Don Johnston Incorporated, must be attached to the Macintosh computer.

Other Methods

When funding for assessment tools is limited, there are other ways to obtain equivalent information from software packages that the clinic has available. Further, freeware and shareware software can be useful and inexpensive. Colorado Easter Seal Society, Don Johnston Incorporated, Edmark, and Mayer-Johnson Company have developed software that can be used to check switch-pressing accuracy and the timing skills necessary for scanning. Resources for software are listed in Appendix B. Therapists may need to keep a pencil-and-paper record of scores and observe the client's ability to interact with the software. Using software that is a teaching tool or game provides a suitable alternative when funds for purchasing evaluation software are limited.

Case Study

ANN

Ann, a 5-year-old girl with mild, ataxic cerebral palsy that affects mainly her right side, was referred to the AT clinic by her primary occupational therapist. The reason for the referral was to determine a more effective method of writing. To be allowed to remain in the mainstream school system and progress to first grade, Ann needed to demonstrate writing skills, that is, writing of her name and all the letters of the alphabet and drawing of simple geometric figures. Ann also needed to be able to cut with scissors. Her mother reported that Ann was using templates to practice making letters and that this activity had been successful in improving Ann's writing ability. However, this was slow, laborious, frustrating, and fatiguing for Ann. Although the teacher wanted Ann to continue practicing printing letters of the alphabet with the rest of the class, she was aware that in the long run, this would not be the first method that Ann would use for completing assignments because she would be slower than the other students.

The team for this assessment consisted of Ann, Ann's mother, the kindergarten teacher, a speech pathologist, and an occupational therapist. The kindergarten teacher brought with her samples of Ann's drawings and printings. Although the child could print, the process was tedious and time consuming. Ann knew her letters and was beginning to learn the standard "qwerty" letter placement on the computer keyboard.

Evaluation

The evaluation began by having Ann sit at a child-sized table and chair. She was able to place her feet flat on the floor. Ann was asked to write her name using a large pencil. She was unable to complete the task, although she was able to draw a recognizable letter "A." When provided with an example, Ann could draw a few letters from the alphabet.

When considering access methods for Ann, it was important to keep in mind the following five factors, which are discussed on page 44:

1. Speed—Which method would she be able to control that would not be slower than the methods her peers were using?
2. Accuracy—Which methods were available that would give her accuracy?

3. Control—Which methods were available that Ann could fully operate?
4. Reliability—Which methods would she be able to access each time?
5. Endurance—Which methods would cause the least amount of fatigue?

Ann was shown several types of pencil aids and holders. In relation to the factors just mentioned, these devices did not adequately provide assistance.

1. Speed—She was still slow in using the pencil.
2. Accuracy—Her letter-printing skills remained poor.
3. Control—The devices did not provide enough additional control over using the pencil to make the writing task less fatiguing or labor intensive.
4. Reliability—She was able to use the devices approximately the same way each time.
5. Endurance—The pencil aids did not decrease her level of fatigue.

An assessment of her skills on a computer keyboard was initiated by the therapist. Macintosh computers were available at Ann's school; thus, the Macintosh keyboard was chosen for the assessment. She was given the Green Dot Test to evaluate her ability to reach all the keys and press one key at a time. She was able to press the six identified keys at a rate of 10 seconds with no errors. Using a keyguard impaired her performance, but using a wrist rest improved it (Table 3–1).

Table 3–1. GREEN DOT TEST

Adaptation to Keyboard	Seconds	Errors
No adaptations	10	0
Keyguard	13	0
Wrist rest	8	0

Ann was also shown the letter location of her name on the keyboard, which she practiced a few times. Although precise measurements of how fast she could write her name were not taken, she could spell her name using the computer more quickly than she could using pencil and paper. Ann was very proud of the way her name looked on the screen; it was neat and in a straight line.

Ann's skills in using the mouse to control the computer were also tested. Mouse skills are critical when using a Macintosh computer. Ann was unable to grasp, simultaneously press the mouse key, and move the mouse (this is called "dragging"). Therefore, the occupational therapist fabricated a handgrip made out of bias tape and fuzzy Velcro. This grip was secured to Ann's right hand and the sticky-back Velcro was secured to the mouse. With this adaptation, Ann placed her hand over the mouse, securing it to her hand with the Velcro. She could then concentrate on the action of pressing the mouse key, allowing her to drag and click the mouse. Without the added burden of maintaining a grip on the mouse, Ann could drag and click without difficulty.

Recommendations

The assessment team recommended that when Ann had assignments involving extensive amounts of writing, she complete her assignment using a computer. For shorter assignments, it was recommended that Ann continue to use handwriting. In this way, she would learn to write the letters of the alphabet and sign her name. In addition, the recommendation was made to the primary occupational therapist that Ann work on fine motor activities to enhance muscle development. This would help improve overall ability to control her muscles when performing fine motor tasks, such as writing.

In summary, use of the keyboard improved Ann's ability to write. She was faster at spelling her name with a keyboard than with paper and pencil. Although Ann was unfamiliar with the keyboard layout, she showed potential for learning the letter arrangement. The assessment team assumed that with practice, her keyboarding skills would improve. Ann had the motor skills needed to control the tool. This method would be reliable in that it would respond the same way every time she pressed the keys. When Ann was seated in a properly fitting child's chair with the keyboard and screen at the proper height, she would be less fatigued than when writing with paper and pencil. Therefore, she would have greater endurance for writing tasks.

Case Study

EVAN

Evan is a 36-year-old bank programmer. He has muscular dystrophy and uses an Everest and Jennings powered wheelchair with a standard joystick control for mobility. Most of his work is done using a computer.

Using the computer, Evan writes simple program codes, updates and maintains databases, and uploads and downloads files between banking sites. To reach all the keys on the computer keyboard, he must change his posture. Evan places his wrists in neutral position and presses the keys with the middle finger of each hand. To reach the keys on the left side, he shifts his entire trunk to the left. To reach the keys on the right side, he must shift his trunk to the right. Continuous shifting of his trunk has become fatiguing for Evan. The keyboard is on a desk that is slightly higher than standard desk height. To reach all the keys, he must lift his arms to rest on the edge of the desk. Lately, it has become more difficult to reach all the keys on the standard keyboard. Evan discussed the problem with his employer. His employer was willing to purchase some equipment for Evan because he found Evan to be a dedicated and valuable employee. Therefore, Evan went to the AT clinic to become acquainted with new technology that might help him with his typing.

Evan explained his problems and goals to the therapist. His basic problem was that the standard keyboard was no longer functional for him. He was experiencing increasing fatigue from using it. Evan's goal was to find a device that would improve his ability to enter commands into the computer so that he could continue working.

Before beginning the evaluation and with Evan's needs specifically in mind, the therapist reviewed the five factors that need to be considered when performing an access assessment:

1. Speed—Evan was slow at typing. The fatigue he was experiencing during the day was contributing to his becoming an even slower typist. Because he needed to accomplish so much work each day, Evan wanted to look for a solution in which he could at least maintain his current typing rate.

2. Accuracy—Accuracy was not a problem for Evan with his current setup; he was fairly accurate with the standard keyboard.

3. Control—Evan needed to be able to control the device. Once he was dropped off by the van service at the front door, he was on his own throughout the day to manage without any help from others. Once the equipment was set up, it needed to be maintenance free.

4. Reliability—Evan was fairly reliable when typing using the standard keyboard.

5. Endurance—Evan was losing some endurance as his disability became exacerbated. He needed technology to help him maintain a certain level of endurance.

First, the therapist showed Evan a small keyboard measuring 4.5 × 7.5 inches. It was not an exact replica of the standard computer keyboard and had fewer keys. It plugged into the parallel port, and special software was needed for the computer to recognize keystrokes. To mimic the standard keyboard keys, some commands required two keystrokes, such as when using the function keys.

In a trial session, Evan used the keyboard for 30 minutes, but the keyboard proved to be unsatisfactory. The contact points for the pressure-sensitive keys did not seem to be evenly distributed. Evan felt that some keys had to be pressed harder than other keys, and at times it was difficult to locate where on the key the contact needed to be made. The therapist encouraged him to take the keyboard to work for 1 week after it was installed on his computer. This way, he could give the keyboard a fair trial and become more accustomed to it than was possible in the 30-minute demonstration session. However, Evan declined the offer. He felt that the 30-minute trial had been enough to get a good feeling for how the keyboard would respond in his office setting.

Next, Evan was shown the Magic Wand keyboard by In Touch Systems (described in Chapter 7). The $3 \times 6\frac{1}{2}$-inch keyboard is a flat metal surface with keys marked on a grid. Two wands attached to the keyboard are used to make contact with the keys. This keyboard had some of the features that Evan had found missing in the other trial keyboard. The Magic Wand was an exact replica of the standard personal computer keyboard, so any keystroke on the Magic Wand would be the same as on a standard PC keyboard. The keyboard plugged into the keyboard port, eliminating the need for software. In addition, there were extra keys on the keyboard that allowed the user to store frequently used words or phrases. Evan found this feature useful because he used some commands frequently when programming. Within a 15-minute training session, Evan was proficient at using this keyboard.

For optimal use, the keyboard was placed in front of Evan at midline on an adjustable table for a 30-minute trial. The table was adjusted so that Even was able to type with his forearms parallel to the floor. Even was able to pick up a wand in each hand and type easily on the keyboard.

After the 30-minute trial, the therapist wanted to confirm Evan's ability to successfully use the keyboard. The therapist gave Evan the Green Dot Test using the standard and the Magic Wand keyboards. The results are displayed in Figure 3–7. After 30 minutes, Evan's typing speed using the Magic Wand keyboard was equivalent to his speed using the standard keyboard. With time, Evan could improve in speed and at least would not decline in speed using the Magic Wand keyboard.

The Magic Wand keyboard eliminated the need for Evan to shift his posture from side to side. After Evan had used the keyboard for 1 week, he was not as fatigued at the end of the day as he was when he used the standard-sized keyboard. Because this keyboard used the key-

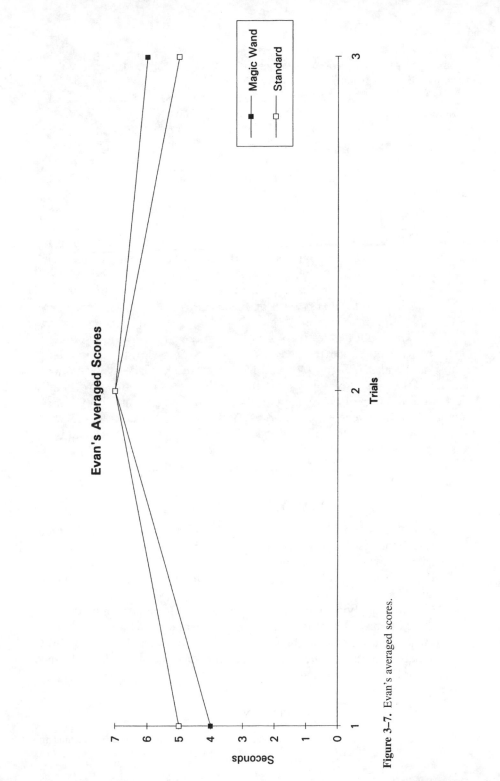

Figure 3–7. Evan's averaged scores.

board port, no additional software was needed. This eliminated the chance of software-conflict problems.

Once the choice of keyboard was determined, the therapist also looked at some of Evan's office furniture. The desk Evan used was too high for typing. After measuring the height of Evan's wheelchair armrest and the table height, the therapist recommended a keyboard drawer. Using a keyboard drawer, Evan could use the armrests on his wheelchair and have his forearm parallel to the floor, obtaining an adequate posture for typing.

Although Evan could easily reach the phone, he had to hold the receiver, a task that was becoming increasingly difficult. The therapist recommended that Evan purchase a telephone handset holder or a speakerphone. Either device eliminated the need for Evan to hold the receiver while he talked on the phone. Evan had a private office; therefore, using a speakerphone would not disturb other workers. Evan chose the speakerphone because of the easy push-button controls and redial feature that came with it.

Working with the AT therapist, Evan discovered ways to continue his employment without fatigue. Evan was satisfied with the devices he chose and with the changes he and his therapist had made at his workstation. Evan's employer was satisfied that Evan could continue working at his normal pace. Both Evan and his employer were satisfied that the devices had been reasonable in price. These changes allowed Evan several additional productive years that he may have lost without the assistance of AT devices.

STUDY QUESTIONS

1. Scanning is considered a more complex form of access than is direct selection. List why and when scanning might be a better choice for some individuals. Be sure to consider the issues discussed in the chapter, such as control of movement, and fatigue or endurance during access.

2. Consider applying the assessments in this chapter to individuals at the extremes of the age range. What adaptations might need to be made to accommodate the strengths and needs of a 3-year-old child? What might need to be done to accommodate the strengths and needs of an elderly individual?

REFERENCES

Angelo, J. (1992). Comparison of three computer scanning modes as an interface method for persons with cerebral palsy. *Journal of Occupational Therapy, 46*(3), 217–222.

Blackstone, S. (1986). *Augmentative communication: An introduction*. Rockville, MD: American Speech-Language-Hearing Association.

Campbell, P. (1985). *Training manual for the training aid*. Wooster, OH: Prentke-Romich.

Cook, A.M. (1988). *The Keyboard Assessment Program*. *Assistive Device Center*. Sacramento, CA: California State University.

Don Johnston Developmental Equipment (1992). *Ke:nx user's manual*. Wauconda, IL: Author.

Don Johnston Incorporated (1984). *Operator's manual for the adaptive firmware card*. Wauconda, IL: Author.

Goosens', C, & Crain, S. (1992). Utilizing switch interfaces with children who are severely physically impaired. Austin, TX: Pro-Ed.

Smith, R.O. (1991). Technology approaches to performance enhancement. In C. Christiansen & C. Baum (Eds.), *Occupational therapy: overcoming human performance deficits*. Thorofare, NJ: Slack Inc.

Yorkston, K., & Carlan, G. (1986). Assessment procedures. In S. Blackstone (Ed.), *Augmentative communication: An introduction*. Rockville, MD: American Speech-Language-Hearing Association.

BIBLIOGRAPHY

Bernstein, L. (Ed.) (1988). *The vocally impaired: Clinical practice and research*. Philadelphia: Grune & Stratton.

LeBanc, M., & Barker, M. (1982). A comparative study of control and display design principles which affect efficient use of communication aids by the severely physically disabled. Final report, Rehabilitation Center. Palo Alto, CA: Children's Hospital at Stanford, Grant No. G008100458.

Smith, R.O. (1992). *Assessment tools for access. Closing the gap*. Minneapolis, MN.

Scanning Modes

There are three basic scanning modes: automatic, inverse, and step. These modes form the foundation of the three basic motor movement patterns used with scanning. The definitions used here are consistent with the operator's manual for the Adaptive Firmware Card (Don Johnston Incorporated, 1984); Goosens' and Crain (1992), and the Ke:nx (Don Johnston Incorporated, 1992).

AUTOMATIC

The user presses the switch; the cursor scans the items in the scanning array automatically. The user presses the switch a second time when the cursor highlights the desired item. Automatic scanning was described in the previous example of spelling the name "David."

INVERSE

The user holds down the switch to activate movement of the cursor across the items. The switch is released when the cursor highlights the desired item. An example of this scanning method can be seen in setting the alarm on a clock radio. One must press the up-arrow button and watch the numbers go by until the desired wake-up time is reached. At the correct moment, the user must release the button to get the correct wake-up time. If the wake-up time is passed, some clock radios will allow the user to go backward. Other clock radios require that the user continue pressing the button while all the numbers flash by until the desired wake-up time is displayed. Without a certain amount of motor control to continue pressing the correct button on the clock radio and reliable motor control to release the button at the correct time, this action is difficult to perform.

STEP

The cursor advances one item with each switch press until the desired item is reached. The absence of a switch press indicates the desired item. A common example is that of moving between two favorite radio stations on the car radio. When the radio is tuned to station A, the up-arrow button must be pressed six times to reach the next favorite station, station B. If the button is pressed only five times, the incorrect station is tuned in. Thus, in step scanning, the switch must be pressed multiple times to skip over the unwanted items. The advantage of step scanning is that anticipation of switch pressing is eliminated. The cursor moves only after the user has pressed the switch. The disadvantage is that the necessity of pressing the switch to move to each item has the potential of causing fatigue.

SCANNING PATTERNS

Several patterns have been developed to increase the scanning speed. Any of the scanning modes can be used; however, the automatic mode is used in the examples throughout this book.

LINEAR OR CIRCULAR

When using a linear or circular pattern (also known as a rotary pattern), the items are scanned one by one. The items are arranged in a vertical line, a horizontal line, or a circle. In the circular form, the indicator may be a picture of a finger, an arrow, a needle, or a light that highlights each item one at a time (Fig. 3–8).

ROW OR COLUMN SCANNING

An entire row of items is highlighted at once, instead of one item at a time. When the row containing the desired item is reached, the user presses the switch indicating that the desired item is in that row. Subsequently, each item in the row is highlighted individually. To type the "H" for the word "Hello," the user activates the scanning device (Fig. 3–9A), waits until the second row of letters is highlighted, and presses the switch to indicate that the desired letter is in the second row (Fig. 3–9B). The user waits until the

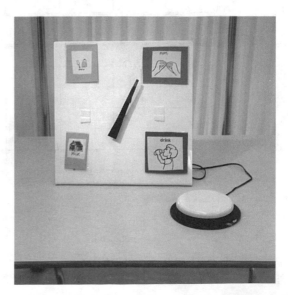

Figure 3–8. Circular scanner.

A	B	C	D	E	F
G	H	I	J	K	L
M	N	O	P	Q	R
S	T	U	V	W	X
Y	Z				

A

A	B	C	D	E	F
G	H	I	J	K	L
M	N	O	P	Q	R
S	T	U	V	W	X
Y	Z				

B

A	B	C	D	E	F
G	H	I	J	K	L
M	N	O	P	Q	R
S	T	U	V	W	X
Y	Z				

C

A	B	C	D	E	F
G	H	I	J	K	L
M	N	O	P	Q	R
S	T	U	V	W	X
Y	Z				

D

H

E

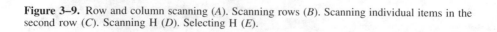

Figure 3–9. Row and column scanning (*A*). Scanning rows (*B*). Scanning individual items in the second row (*C*). Scanning H (*D*). Selecting H (*E*).

letter "H" is highlighted and presses the switch again to indicate that this is the desired letter (Fig. 3–9C–D). The letter "H" is displayed on the screen (Fig. 3–9E).

FREQUENCY SCANNING

Another method used to increase scanning speed is the arrangement of the icons or letters on the display. The letters or symbols are arranged by frequency of use. Those letters or symbols used most frequently are placed in the scanning array so that the cursor highlights them first. Letters or symbols used infrequently are at the end of the display. This saves time as the user prepares communication or written documents. An example of a scanning array set up for row or column scanning using the most frequently used letters is shown in Figure 3–10.

DIRECTED SCANNING

The cursor is directed by the user's moving a joystick. The control is much like that of a video game, where the object is to move in a given direction to reach a goal. If the joystick is moved in the forward position, the cursor moves upward on the screen. If the joystick is moved to the left, the cursor also moves left. One of two methods is used to indicate the desired item: an additional switch or an automatic entry. With the first method, the individual indicates a choice by pressing the extra switch. In this method, an incorrect item is rarely chosen. Using automatic entry, the user places the cursor on the item of choice and waits a predetermined amount of time to indicate this choice. As the user uses the joystick to highlight the desired item for a predetermined length of time, it is displayed on the screen. Properly choosing the acceptance time is important and can be a frustrating process. Trial-and-error problem solving may be helpful in finding an appropriate acceptance time. This type of scanning typically provides quicker access than the other methods described but requires more motor control.

I	O	T	E	A	N
H	S	M	D	Y	R
U	L	W	F	G	B
C	K	P	V	J	X
Z	Q				

Figure 3–10. Letter arrangement according to frequency of use.

Resources for Commercially Available Software Packages

Colorado Easter Seal Society
Center for Adapted Technology
   Catalog
5755 West Alameda Ave.
Lakewood, CO 80226-3500
303-233-1666

Don Johnston Incorporated
1000 N. Rand Rd., Bldg. 115
PO Box 639
Wauconda, IL 60084-0639
1-800-999-4660

Edmark
PO Box 3218
Redmond, VA 98073-3218
1-800-362-2890

Mayer-Johnson Company
PO Box 1579
Solana Beach, CA 92075-1579
619-550-0084

Scanning Assessment Tool
Product Information
Occupational Therapy
University at Buffalo
515 Kimball Tower
Buffalo, NY 14214
716-829-3141

CHAPTER 4

SWITCHES

Assistive Technology Guide

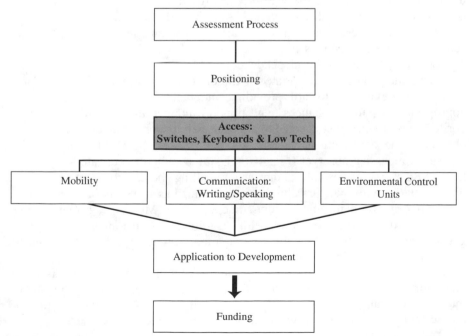

USING SWITCHES WITH DEVICES AND TOYS
Rationale for Switch Use

Children with physical disabilities often find exploration and environmental control difficult, if not impossible. Typically, children begin to explore the environment beyond their reach by 9 or 10 months (with the onset of crawling and creeping), but children with physical disabilities are limited or prevented from doing so by their physical limitations. For young children with disabilities, using toys with switches can assist in exploration and control of the environment in the context of play. Play is the child's work and thus an appropriate area in which to initiate exploration skills. Furthermore, using toys with switches can be viewed as preliminary to operating environmental control units, powered wheelchairs, and augmentative communication devices (Musselwhite, 1986).

Likewise, adults with physical disabilities have difficulty controlling aspects of their environment. They may not be able to turn down the lights, move from place to place, or operate the compact disc (CD) player or television. Switches can assist individuals in gaining or regaining control over these devices. This chapter explores the uses, characteristics, and mountings of switches. This information will assist therapists as they evaluate which switches may be appropriate for a particular individual.

The therapist should review the type of activities that are appropriate for the cognitive and motor skill developmental levels prior to developing an intervention plan. Knowing the appropriate level of activities for the individual being assessed assists the therapist in providing successful sessions and peaking the interests of that individual. Activities that are too easy may bore the individual, whereas activities that are too difficult may contribute to a sense of failure and helplessness. The individual may then refuse future activities that could improve independence.

Activities that are appropriate for the client's developmental and motor-skill level are a step toward providing independence. For children, age-appropriate toys and appliances (e.g., popcorn popper, tape recorder with favorite songs or stories) connected to a switch help the children learn to control objects in the environment and allow others to see the child as a "doer" instead of a passive observer (Fig. 4–1). Using a switch to activate a toy may be a child's first successful attempt at controlling the environment (Musselwhite, 1986). With switch technology, the child has a means of controlling his or her environment and gaining independence. Moreover, research has demonstrated that young children with disabilities spend longer periods engaged in an activity with toys that react compared with toys that do not react (Bambara, Spiegel-McGill, Shores, & Fox, 1984).

For adults, the rationale for using single-switch access methods is that other input devices, such as keyboards, have been unsatisfactory, too labor intensive, or fraught with errors. Usually, adults are looking for ways to increase their independence at work, at home, and in recreational pursuits.

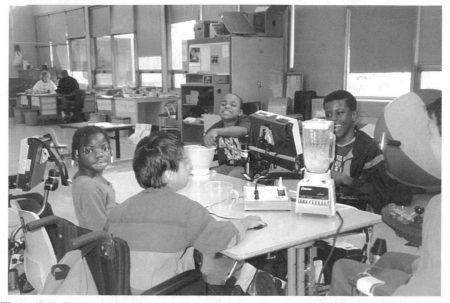

Figure 4–1. Children engaged in an activity using a switch to operate an electric blender.

Purpose for Switch Use

For children, the following are typical purposes of using switches:

- Teach cause and effect
- Teach children how to independently engage in activities
- Provide methods for the children to participate in group activities
- Give children control over a component of their environment

Teach Cause and Effect

Children usually develop the basic concept of cause and effect very early. Developmental texts indicate that by 8 months of age, the infant has learned "if I cry, Mama comes," and a little later, they learn "if I shake this rattle, it makes a noise." The ability to affect the environment helps develop the child's sense of control over it and develops the child's understanding of the fact that a particular action will cause a predictable consequence. For this concept to develop in children with disabilities, the environment needs to be arranged so that the child has opportunities to effectively interact with it. The first switch interaction usually involves the child's repeating the same movement (e.g., repeatedly pressing a switch connected to a toy or tape recorder) to obtain a consistent response. In this way, children learn that their actions can be meaningful and that they can control some activity in their immediate environment. Helping children learn to control their movements in a purposeful manner is critical to learning cause and effect. In addition, understanding basic cause and effect forms a necessary foundation for more so-phisticated environmental interactions.

Teach Children How to Independently Engage in Activities

Many times, children with severe disabilities develop learned helpless-ness (Goosens' & Crain, 1992). There are so many activities in which they are unable to engage that some children learn to wait and allow others to perform the activity for them while they watch. Other children use disruptive behaviors as a means of gaining control. Switch technology increases the possibilities of purposeful interactions with objects in the environment. Using toys in conjunction with technology begins to narrow the gap between what the child can and cannot do. For instance, with a switch, the child can run a popcorn popper and make popcorn for the rest of the class, be in charge of a buzzer to start and stop games and relay races, or play computer games alone or with several other players. Switch technology allows the child to take a more active role in educational and recreational activities.

Provide Methods for Children to Participate in Group Activities

Toys or appliances with switches can be used as tools to create an en-vironment in which children with disabilities are able to participate in group activities. For example, cars in a toy train set are filled with snacks for every child in the group. The children are grouped so that the train cars are within their reach. The child with a disability can then be in charge of pressing the switch connected to the toy train. As the child presses and releases the switch, the toy train stops in front of each child in the group. Each child takes his or her snack, and then the child with the disability presses the switch again to move the train to the next child. Use of toys in this manner (such as bringing food or objects to others) builds on cause and effect and begins the process of learning to operate a tool.

Give Children Control Over a Component of Their Environment

Toys with switches are part of a larger plan to help children overcome physical limitations and act on their environment at their development level. Examples include using a battery-operated toy car to knock down a tower; taping a felt-tip marker to a toy car, placing the car on a sheet of drawing paper, and having the child press the switch to "draw" on the paper; and using a tape recorder so everyone can sing songs or play musical chairs. Toys with switches are a preliminary step to introducing children to methods of accessing other forms of assistive technology (AT), such as computers for schoolwork, augmentative communication devices for enhanced communication, and environmental control units for controlling televisions, telephones, and the temperature. The purpose of introducing the use of switch-activated toys is *not* to have the child watch a toy bear dance or a dog bark, but to make a much bigger impact on the developing child's life.

For adults, the purposes of single-switch use are similar to those described for children. Adults may begin with single switches as a means of providing greater independence. Based on the goals established by the adult or the adult's caregiver, single-switch use may be the first step toward independence in written or spoken communication, control of a wheelchair, or control of environmental devices. As with the child, the switch activation is not the goal or highest level of switch skill attainable. However, it is a place to begin.

One of the devices that adults may desire to control is a computer. Switches can be used for games, word processors, and other software programs. Single-switch telephone dialers can keep people connected to others outside their home. One example of this is a man with multiple sclerosis using a single switch to answer and place telephone calls. Using this device, his wife can continue working. She can call him several times during her working hours to talk to him, and he can call her, his friends, and emergency numbers by using a chin switch connected to a telephone dialer. Single switches can also be used to operate radios and CD players to enable individuals with head injuries to engage in activities they enjoyed prior to being injured.

HOW SWITCHES WORK

A switch is basically a simple electrical connection. Presented here is a description of how switches work and how they are connected to standard battery-operated toys or other devices. Understanding fundamental functions of switches helps clarify the potential of a switch for use with AT.

As shown in Figure 4–2, a switch is a simple electrical unit made up of a phone jack, two wires, and two plates. Each wire goes to one of the plates. The plates are the parts of the switch that move when pressed so that contact is made between the two wires. Prior to activation, the two wires do not touch, keeping the electrical circuit open and the toy or device deactivated. When the switch is pressed, the two wires touch, closing the electrical circuit. Electricity then flows from the power supply to the device to make the toy or device operate. When the switch is released, the contact is interrupted, and the device stops.

There are two types of switches, momentary and latching. *Momentary* means that as long as the switch is pressed, the electrical connection is made, and the toy or device is activated as described. The mechanism is similar to that of a drinking fountain. Pressure must be maintained on the bar of the

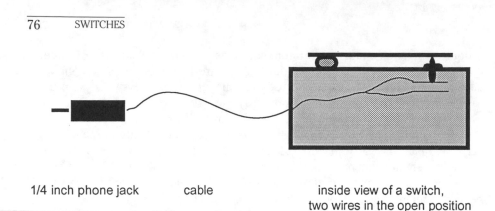

1/4 inch phone jack   cable   inside view of a switch,
                                                     two wires in the open position

Figure 4–2. Anatomy of a switch.

drinking fountain or water does not come out of the spout. Another example is the light on a wristwatch in which pressure must be maintained on the button to illuminate the watch face. Most switches used with toys for children with disabilities are the momentary type of switch. *Latching* means that as the switch is pressed and released, the toy or device remains activated until the switch is pressed again. Examples of latch-type switches include a radio, flashlight, or lamp.

Properties of Switches

Evaluating the properties of switches is necessary when evaluating people with physical disabilities and making switch recommendations. Choosing a switch begins as the therapist or AT team discerns the movements over which the individual has the most control. Ability and the potential switch sites will guide the team as they decide which switch(es) the individual should try using. The following is a description of switch characteristics that must be kept in mind when evaluating the usefulness of switches for particular children. This list pertains primarily to switches that are activated through pressure (Goosens' & Crain, 1992).

Force

Switches differ as to the amount of force needed for activation and are categorized as needing minimal, medium, or heavy force to press. Some switches are activated with minimal force, such as the Plate Switch by Tash or P-Switch by Prentke-Romich Company (PRC). Other switches, such as the Soft Switch by Tash and the Foot Switch by Radio Shack, are designed to endure forceful movements. The Soft Switch provides some protection through a soft cover and foam padding so that individuals are not injured while activating the switch.

One of the main factors to consider when examining the force needed to press a switch is whether the prognosis indicates that the individual will become weaker. In this case, switches that require minimum force should be presented to prevent fatigue and conserve energy. In contrast, when the individual has many extraneous movements, a switch that requires minimal force can be frustrating because he or she may be pressing the switch unintentionally and possibly drawing unwanted attention to himself or herself by activating an augmentative communication device when it is inappropriate. In this case, a switch requiring more force to press is more practical and less frustrating. The individual will have more control over such a switch, activating it only when desired.

Most commercially available switches are not designed so that force can be changed. However, there is one exception. The amount of force needed to activate the Foot Switch can be easily changed. This is accomplished by changing the springs, cutting off a section of the springs, or exchanging them for weaker springs (Goosens' & Crain, 1992). Scott-Taplin (1988) provides a description of the amount of force needed for a number of widely used switches.

Feedback

Feedback notifies the individual when he or she has activated the switch. Without feedback, the individual may not know if he or she is making the correct movement or needs to adjust the movement to activate the switch (Goosens' & Crain, 1992). The absence of feedback can be frustrating to the child or adult as he or she tries to activate the toy or device. There are several types of feedback, including auditory, visual, tactile, and kinesthetic (Goosens' & Crain, 1992). Each one is discussed separately.

Auditory

Most switches provide an audible click when pressed. This lets the individual know that the proper movement has been made and that the switch should begin activating the device to which it is attached. Auditory feedback becomes increasingly important when switch placement is located out of the individual's visual field (i.e., around the head, near the knee or foot, or underneath a lap tray, where vision is occluded). When the individual cannot see the switch or the body part that comes into contact with the switch, an auditory click is important.

Visual

Some switches are equipped with a small light that is illuminated when the switch is activated. This provides visual feedback. Obviously, the light must be in a position where the individual can view it, or this feature is not useful. Switches with lights are particularly helpful to individuals with hearing impairments and people spending time in libraries and concert or lecture halls. Additionally, visual feedback is useful for individuals who do not wish to draw attention to themselves, such as students in classroom settings.

Tactile

The surfaces of some switches are rich in tactile feedback. These materials are helpful in locating the switch for children with blindness or impaired vision. Examples are the Soft Switch from both Tash and Crestwood and the Petite Pillow Switch from Toys for Special Children. Each of these switches has a velvety fabric cover. The Treadle Switch by Tash and the Foot Switch by Radio Shack provide a rough surface. Slick plastic switches that provide little feedback can be covered with a variety of materials to increase the sensation. Materials such as a rough or soft fabric, one with a nubby surface, or an upholstery material, burlap, or sandpaper all provide additional tactile feedback. In addition, this technique is useful when two or more switches are to be used. Using a different covering on each switch helps to clearly identify each switch.

Some switches vibrate to let the user know that the switch is activated. Vibration may be an alternative to auditory feedback. An example of this type of switch can be found in the Vibrating Pillow Switch by Toys for Special Children.

Kinesthetic

When switches require some force for activation, the user receives kinesthetic feedback resulting from the movement. Minimal kinesthetic input is received when there are no moving parts or when the switch is activated by minimal touch. Kinesthetic feedback provides important cues. It helps individuals with an impaired proprioceptive sense to know if they pressed the switch with enough pressure to activate it or if they need to apply more force. Switches that provide limited kinesthetic feedback are classified as pressure (touch) sensitive and may be difficult for some people to use effectively.

Travel

Travel is the distance the switch must be pushed before it is activated. Switches range from pressure- (touch-) sensitive switches that have no travel to wobble and leaf switches that travel a few centimeters before being activated. Switches that travel are inappropriate for people who experience pain when they move, such as those with arthritis. Switches that travel may be appropriate for those who have gross motor control and poor fine motor control. They use a gross motor movement to attempt switch activation, generally with successful results.

Size

The size of switches can vary a great deal. Switches used for children are usually bigger in diameter to help the child locate the switch. As children develop skill and mature, it may be more aesthetically pleasing to provide smaller switches that are not as noticeable and do not look as childish. Due to motor control limitations, decreasing the size of the switch with increasing age is not always possible. Dark-colored switches can be used for adults who continue to need a large switch but do not want to draw attention to it. Additionally, large switches are at times used with adults at the beginning of training and then replaced with smaller switches as their control for activation improves.

Another factor that must be considered with size is the height of the switch (Goosens' & Crain, 1992). Height is particularly important when the switch is positioned on the lap tray and requires the individual to raise his or her hand (from a resting position) in an upward direction, move over and above the switch, and then place it on top of the switch for activation. Although this task does not sound monumental, it can be difficult for individuals with severe disabilities to execute, particularly when scanning and a timing element are involved. If the switch appears to be appropriate but is too high, it may be necessary to cut a hole in the lap tray and recess the switch into the tray to avoid the additional movements of raising the hand up and over the switch. Another solution is to place the hands on a built-up surface and the switch on the lap tray. Using this position, the individual needs to drop the hand over the switch. This eliminates the up, over, and down procedure previously described.

Weight

Weight is usually not an issue when the switch is mounted to the wheelchair or lap tray (Goosens' & Crain, 1992). Weight becomes an issue when the switch is mounted to be freestanding. An example is using a switch on a mount that is fastened to the wheelchair only at one point. It may be in jeopardy of swaying as the chair is propelled, or moving from the desired location as the day progresses. In a freestanding mount, the weight of the switch can pull it out of reach. Another situation occurs when the switch is to be mounted on the individual. Excessive weight can affect energy level and can adversely affect posture, as could occur with a light pointer on the side of the head for a small child.

Moisture Resistance

Switches used around the mouth or on top of a lap tray must be sealed to protect them against saliva and food spillage. Moisture and the collection of food particles can decrease the life of the switch, prevent activation, and cause rust to form in the working parts.

Multiple Switches

Some switches are physically joined. For instance, to allow individuals to operate an environmental control unit and wheelchair, the switches for both may be in one housing unit. Examples of such switches include the Push-Button Control by Zygo, the Wafer by Tash (five membrane switches in one low-profile housing), the Penta by Tash (a five-button switch), the Star by Tash (a five-button switch in the configuration of a plus sign), the Arm Slot Control Switch by PRC, and the Arm Slot Switch Controller by APT Technology Inc., formerly known as Du-It Controls Systems Group. One disadvantage of such switches is that they do not permit flexibility in determining the proper placement for each of the five switch sites. They are fixed in a particular arrangement. Another disadvantage is that the switches are a fixed distance apart from one another. If this distance is too far or too close for an individual to press, then separate switches need to be considered. An advantage of this arrangement is that the switches do not get out of position from each other and are easier to maintain as a whole.

Safety

Switches must be reviewed for safety. They must not have sharp edges that could cause injury or come apart easily to expose sharp edges. They also must be mounted so that body parts (the head or arm) cannot get caught underneath them.

Several types of switches are available that incorporate many of the properties discussed. When evaluating switch access and switch type, it is important to have a variety on hand for trial. It is usually advisable to have at least one switch that represents each of the switch characteristics. Resources for purchasing switches are listed in the Appendices.

CUSTOM-FABRICATED SWITCHES

Switches can be custom fabricated, meaning made by the therapist, parent, teacher, or technician. Although in the short term this may appear to be a less expensive approach, in the long term it is usually not advisable. A major consideration in deciding whether to purchase or make a switch is cost. If a therapist spends his or her time making switches, the cost must be calculated based on the time, overhead, and materials required in fabrication. A switch requiring 1½ hours of a therapist's time is not likely to be a less expensive item than one available commercially. In addition, the therapist may not be able to directly charge for the time he or she spent in switch making, causing either the therapist or the facility to bear the cost of the custom-fabricated construction. A second factor to consider is that custom-fabricated switches tend to break more easily than do commercially available switches. The casing or connection is usually not as strong and may not be able to take the wear and abuse that commercially available switches are built to withstand. Third, custom-fabricated switches are not as reliable as commercially available switches. The mechanism inside the switch that activates a toy or other device may not always connect reliably. This means that the client does not know if he or she has pressed hard enough, if he or she has missed the switch, or if the switch is malfunctioning. This can be frustrating during training periods. Fourth, the individual who fabricated the switch is liable for the safety of the switch. If the switch has rough edges or sharp corners that cause an injury to the client or another person, the fabricator may be liable for the injury. Finally, when the switch malfunctions, the user will return it to the therapist for repairs. Given the busy schedule kept by therapists, it is likely that a repair request will come at an inopportune time. Commercially available switches come with a warranty for this type of situation. Further, commercially available switches can be kept in stock for such problems or they can be ordered. The switch can be replaced easily with minimal interference with the therapist's busy schedule.

SWITCH MOUNTING

Two categories of mounting options are available: temporary for assessments and permanent for frequent use. Mountings ideal for assessing the individual's switch-pressing abilities are commercially available in two styles: ready-to-use mountings and kits. Permanent mountings are available commercially as ready-to-assemble style kits or as custom fabricated. Switches are generally mounted to something in the environment, the wheelchair, the lap tray, the table, or the individual's body.

Mountings Used During Assessments

When evaluating the optimal mounting placement for switch access, the switch needs to be placed in several different positions as the AT team works to discover the individual's strengths and weaknesses. During this evaluation period, it is important to have a mounting device that allows the AT team to change the switch position quickly and then hold that position so that it is sturdy yet temporary. This mounting device can also be sent home with the individual on a temporary basis so that he or she can practice activating the switch while it is in a particular position. This helps ensure that the optimal switch mounting position has been found.

Mounts used in the assessment process are camera mounts, gooseneck structures, and assessment kits. These mounting systems allow the AT team to easily move the switch into positions that appear to be optimal for switch placement. Adjustments to the camera mount are made by changing the position of the arms of the mount by tightening and loosening the lever. For the gooseneck, the mount is manually moved into position. Camera mounts are available from AbleNet (Universal Switch Mounting System and Slim Armstrong) (Fig. 4–3). Gooseneck types of mounts are available from Crestwood, PRC, and Tash. Both mounting options are easy to clamp onto a wheelchair or table and adjust quickly during assessments.

Switch mounting kits provide a variety of parts that are connected together in innumerable combinations to achieve the optimal switch position for the individual. Some of the switch mounting kits available are the Switch

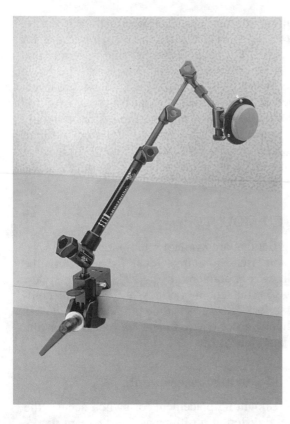

Figure 4–3. Slim Armstrong Mount. (Courtesy of AbleNet, Inc., Minneapolis, MN.)

Mounting Kit from Tash and the Adaptive Fixtures Kit from Zygo (Fig. 4–4). The kits include clamps, rods, tubes, and gooseneck arms.

Permanent Mounting Fixtures

Generally, several people are involved in the lives of individuals with disabilities. Obtaining the proper switch placement may be difficult if the switch must be remounted following caretaking or other activities. Therefore, once the proper switch position has been found, a permanent type of mount is advisable. This is particularly critical for individuals who use a switch that is occluded from vision, such as a switch placed at the side of the head, by the leg or foot, or underneath a lap tray. If the switch is not placed in exactly the same position each time, the individual may have difficulty locating it. This may occur every time the individual gets out of the wheelchair. Therefore, precision in switch placement is of great concern.

Permanent mounting systems are commercially available or can be custom fabricated. Custom-fabricated mounting systems may be used when nothing else works and when technical help is available. The commercially available kits were discussed previously in the chapter; however, a few additional comments are presented here.

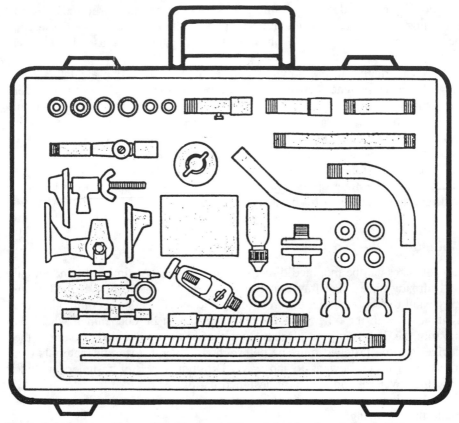

Figure 4–4. Adaptive Fixtures Kit. (Courtesy of Zygo Industries, Inc., Portland, OR.)

Gooseneck mounts discussed previously can be permanent. This works well if the input device is a microphone, and the individual does not actually come into contact with the mounting system, thereby putting pressure on it. Goosenecks quickly move out of position if the individual generates a great deal of force during switch activation. This is a frustrating situation and can be avoided by using a different type of permanent mounting structure for individuals who generate such heavy force during switch activation.

Switch mounting systems developed from kits can also become permanent switch mounting solutions. Thus, kits can be used in two ways. The parts taken from the kit and used for a particular mount can be the permanent mount and sent home with the client. The parts used can be ordered or several extra parts can be kept on hand so the evaluation kit is restocked when items have been used from it. Alternatively, the mount configuration can be noted and the necessary parts ordered (Zygo Industries, 1995).

A custom-fabricated mounting option may consist of chlorinated poly-vinyl chloride (CPVC) pipe fitted together (Goosens' & Crain, 1992). The CPVC pipe can be mounted directly to the wheelchair and painted to match the upholstery. For children, perfect fits can be made by cutting the pipe and additional pieces added as the child grows. Many technology service delivery programs provide custom mounting as part of their AT services. These can be as simple as using Velcro on a lap tray or as complex as fabricating a metal hardware mount.

An alternative to the previous permanent system is one available from Zygo for lever switches activated with a head motion. This system allows for the switch to be swung out of the way without losing the proper position. One or two switches, one on either side of the head, can be used with this system. This system is most stable and accurate when two rods are used, one on either side of the chair.

Thus far, all the mounting options discussed have attached to the wheelchair. Other mounting options must be discussed: attachment to the lap tray and bed and attachment to the body.

Mounting to the Lap Tray

Devices can be mounted directly to the lap tray. At times, the individual will already have a lap tray that can be used. At other times, the AT team may want to recommend a different lap tray that will better accommodate the switch. As with the other assessments, it must first be determined where on the tray the device will be placed. Once that has been decided, then how the device is to be fastened must be determined. Several different materials can be used to fasten devices to lap trays. Different types of fasteners include poly lock, Velcro, and specially designed hardware.

Questions to keep in mind during assessment for lap tray mounting include the following:

1. Does the individual need this lap tray space for other activities? Does he or she eat, draw, and read in this same space? If the answer is yes, then the device must be fastened with something that is removable so that the other activities can take place.
2. Can the lap tray be removed with the device on it, or does the device make it too heavy?
3. Is the device attached to an external power source plugged into a wall outlet? If the user decides to move, will the device, mount, or switch be damaged?
4. Does the device need to stay in one environment or move between environments?
5. How permanent will this device be? Will the individual be obtaining a different device soon?
6. Does excess moisture from food or saliva cause a concern that needs to be addressed?

Answering these questions helps avoid device placement that is not practical in all environments. Proper mounting works in harmony with the other activities in which the individual engages throughout the day.

Mounting to the Body

Mounting a switch to the body usually involves switches that are sensitive to small muscle movements. This type of mounting is recommended when the individual's muscle control is limited to one or two isolated muscle groups, or the condition is one in which the individual will become weaker. Examples of body-mounted switches include the P-Switch (PRC), Infrared/Sound/Touch (IST) Switch (Words+), Eyebrow Switch (Words+), Mercury Switch (Crestwood), Chin Switch (PRC), SCI Chin Controller (APT Technology Inc., formerly known as Du-It Controls Systems Group), and SCI Tongue/Lip Controller (APT Technology Inc., formerly known as Du-It Controls Systems Group). The P-Switch and Mercury Switch are mounted to the body with straps to hold them in place; the Infrared Switch can be mounted to eyeglass frames or a baseball cap. The Eyebrow Switch is mounted to a baseball cap. The mount for the Chin Switch and SCI Chin Controller attaches to the chest. The mount for the SCI Tongue/Lip Controller attaches to the head similar to a head pointer.

Securing the Mount

Mounting should blend and not attract attention. When deciding how to mount a switch, it is important to keep several principles in mind.

Support Other Activities

The mounting system should not interfere with activities of daily living, such as transfers, feeding, or bathroom activities. The mount may need to come off, swing away, or support other functions that need to be carried out during the day. This must be considered at the time of recommendation and construction. The mount should easily snap into place. If the mount has "play" in it or needs to be adjusted every time it is to be positioned, the people who will be positioning it throughout the day will probably do so with some variability. Thus, the switch will be in a less than ideal position, making it difficult for the individual to find and press it. This problem is magnified when the switch is out of the individual's visual range.

Aesthetically Pleasing

Mounts should blend in with their surroundings. If they are to be mounted to the lap tray, they should not detract from seeing the individual. Tubing fastened to the wheelchair can be painted the same color as the upholstery or painted a color chosen by the client.

KNOW YOUR BATTERIES

When using battery-operated toys and equipment, it is important to know the differences between batteries to obtain the best usage and spend resources wisely. It is important to be aware of some of the basic differences in batteries, because this understanding increases the longevity of the devices in which the batteries are used.

Battery Types

Batteries are either rechargeable (nickel-cadmium) or disposable. Rechargeable batteries are more economical over time. Initial costs may seem high because the recharger will need to be purchased, and the batteries are more expensive than nonrechargeable ones; however, replacement costs are not incurred. Thus, using rechargeable batteries is cost-effective. However, rechargeable batteries are not without problems, because they need recharging. A single charge on a rechargeable battery does not last as long as a disposable battery. As such, if a battery is to be used for a long time, as when using a flashlight, the rechargeable battery may not be the best choice. When rechargeable batteries are left in a device that is used only once in a while, by the time it is needed again, the rechargeable batteries could need recharging. Further, rechargeable batteries quit suddenly, giving no warning that they are running low on power. Therefore, batteries need to be recharged before they are completely drained. This means that recharging must become part of the daily routine. It is frustrating to encourage a child's participation in an activity only to have that child wait as the therapist searches for batteries that are still active. A session with a child could just be beginning, and the toy the child is excited about using may suddenly stop working, leaving the therapist using precious therapy time to search for active batteries. To solve these difficulties, it is important when using rechargeable batteries to keep in the clinic at least two sets of batteries in sizes most commonly used in the toys and devices. One set should be in the toy(s) or device(s), and the other should be in the recharger.

Disposable batteries consist of two types: alkaline and zinc chloride. Alkaline batteries cost more but last longer than either zinc chloride or rechargeable batteries. Both alkaline and zinc chloride batteries lose their power slowly when compared with rechargeable batteries. This gives the therapist, parent, guardian, or attendant time to replace them before they are completely discharged.

Battery Hints

Do not combine different name brands or new and old batteries. This drains the newer, stronger battery. Store batteries in a cool, dry place because heat will shorten their life. If particular toys will not be used for a long time, such as over the summer in a school setting, remove the batteries. Batteries can corrode and ruin the device if left in the battery compartment for long periods. All batteries need clean, shiny contact surfaces to work efficiently.

If the battery case becomes encrusted with grime, a cotton swab with alcohol or baking soda works well to clean it.

At times, toys will work too well with new batteries. They either are too fast or produce too many actions, sounds, and sights. By experimenting with the toys, some of these actions can be slowed or discontinued. To do this, cut a dowel rod the same size as the battery. Insert two thumb tacks, one in each end, into the dowel. Then insert the dowel into the battery compartment in place of one of the batteries. For some toys, the placement of the dowel in the battery compartment will affect the functions of the toy. At other times, the number of dowels used in the battery compartment affects the functions. An example is a toy dog that barks and flips over. By placing one dowel in the battery compartment, the dog does not bark but continues to flip over. Another example is a train. The train moves and has a light and whistle. By strategically placing a dowel in place of one battery, the whistle or light can be disconnected. This strategy is helpful for children who are overstimulated by too many actions happening at once.

LEARNING SWITCH CONTROL

When developing therapy sessions for switch control, the therapist will often want to create an environment that encourages a certain motor pattern. The therapist should set up situations when this motor pattern is used repeatedly to gain improved control over the particular movement. This helps the individual understand what movement he or she needs to make to control the device. The movements that the therapist will usually want the individual to practice are switch pressing, switch holding, and switch releasing. Successful teaching sessions for these skills depend on age-appropriate toys or devices and the positive reinforcement obtained through the switch press. Switch latching devices can facilitate the switch-use training process.

Switch Latching Device

A latching device allows a momentary switch to be used as if it were a latching switch. The switch is connected to the latching device, and the latching device is connected to the toy. Once the connection is made, the switch can be released, but the electrical circuit is not broken. Latching devices are available for battery-operated toys or devices and electrical devices. The following are examples of ways to use switch latching devices to teach specific skills. Many of these examples are directed toward children. Cognitively intact adults will practice these skills until they have reached mastery once they understand the reasons behind practice. Children may need additional motivation to maintain a high level of involvement. Using the switch latching device, the therapist can develop games and activities for switch pressing training.

Switch Pressing

The therapist will want children or adults to practice switch pressing if they have difficulty maintaining enough pressure on a switch once it has been pressed. During practice sessions, the therapist should reward even the smallest ability to press the switch. The child may become discouraged at being able to activate the toy only momentarily. This scenario can happen when using a momentary switch. The switch latching device can change this experience by maintaining the closed circuit for a predetermined length of time so that the toy continues to be activated, even though the child has released the switch.

To encourage multiple switch activations, or to assist a child who has difficulty maintaining contact with a switch, a timer on the switch latching device should be set. The timer allows the toy to remain activated for a predetermined length of time once the child has pressed the switch. This feature is useful when the therapist wants the individual to practice the new motor skill of switch pressing. For children who are learning switch pressing and have difficulty maintaining pressure on the switch, the latching device will maintain the closed loop circuit so that the toy continues to operate without maintaining pressure on the switch. The time can be set so that after 2 seconds or an appropriate length of time, the toy stops, and the child must press the switch again so that the toy will play. Several switch pressings can be practiced within one therapy session.

Switch Holding

Switch holding allows the individual to activate the toy or device only after he or she has successfully held the switch down for a specified amount of time. Such holding is an important skill to practice when preparing for scanning. With scanning, the individual must continuously press the switch while the cursor moves to the desired item. This motion is also used in inverse scanning. To practice holding, the timer on the switch latching device is set so that the toy or device is not activated until the switch has been pressed for a given amount of time.

Switch Releasing

If switch release is the desired movement, the switch latch device is set so that the toy or device is activated only when the switch is pressed and released. This motion is important in inverse scanning and, once learned, may be useful for other activities.

Switch latching devices are sold by several companies. Although latching devices do not have identical features, the main ones are described here. AbleNet sells a Switch Latch and Timer. The timer allows the therapist to set the length of time the "latch" maintains the electrical connection. They also make Power Link, the latching device for electrical appliances. Toys for Special Children makes individual latching devices, each performing one function, and a Universal Module, which combines many of these features into one unit. One module counts the number of switch closures made; one reverses the action needed (i.e., if the switch normally must be kept pressed to activate the toy, when using this module, the switch must be released for the toy to activate). A time module controls the amount of time the switch will activate the toy. Push on/Push off allows the switch to activate the toy with the first press and turn the toy off with the second switch press, and Rhythm Generator controls the speed at which the toy operates. Toys for Special Children's "AND" module requires the user(s) to press two switches before the toy can be activated. This is designed for cooperative play and teaching motor control of two body parts. It is a multiswitch module for turn taking. Tash makes the Switch Latch and the Dual Switch Latch. The Dual Switch Latch allows two switches to be used independently for two devices. Thus, the choice of latching device depends on the needs of the client. Addresses for these companies are in the Appendices.

ADAPTERS

Usually, switches are made with a standard ⅛-inch plug and switch-ready toys come fitted with ⅛-inch jacks. Unfortunately, switch plugs have not been standardized. Some toys and switches use phone plugs (¼ inch) or subminiature phone plugs (³⁄₃₂ inch). When a toy or switch has a jack or plug of a different size, an adapter can be used with the switch. Several adapters should be kept on hand so that there is no disruption in the activity being presented. In some clinics, the adapter is left on the toy; in other clinics, the adapters are kept together. Adapters can be purchased at electronics stores, such as Radio Shack.

Case Study

ERIC

Eric is a 6-year-old boy who attends public school and has cerebral palsy. He uses a powered wheelchair for mobility, which is equipped with a wooden lap tray. Eric has more control over his right hand than his left. There is tightness in Eric's left elbow joint. He tends to keep the left arm close to his body and does not use it functionally. At times, Eric places his left hand underneath the lap tray for stability. Currently, he uses his right fist to point to the letters or words on his communication board. The squares on the communication board are 2 × 2 inches.

Eric's teacher is encouraging Eric's spelling skills to increase the number of subjects he can discuss. Eric has no method of permanently storing messages with his current communication system. Generally, it is difficult for his teacher and parents to be certain what letter or word Eric is pointing to, due to his erratic arm movements. Often the listener must guess the desired letter, with Eric indicating through body gestures whether the listener has guessed correctly. This process can be laborious and lengthy for Eric and the listener as well as tiring for Eric.

Eric was evaluated for an augmentative communication device and writing system to help him keep up in his studies at school. The assessment by the AT team determined that at this time, Eric was not a candidate for using direct selection as an input method, due to his inability to isolate a finger movement. Also, if he were to use his fist for direct selection, he would be able to fit only a few symbols on a communication board. The AT team also decided that Eric's right hand and head movement needed further investigation before the most optimal switch type and position were established.

Eric was asked to activate a toy for assessing switch use. Eric fully grasped the concept of cause and effect. His mother told the therapist that he was very fond of bubbles. Therefore, the activity chosen was pressing a switch connected to a small fan. When he activated the fan, his mother held a bubble wand dipped in bubble solution in front of the fan. The bubbles were directed at any individual Eric chose. Eric was motivated to learn how to press the switch to make bubbles. Bombarding people with bubbles was very motivating for Eric.

The AT team's initial efforts focused on the use of Eric's right fisted hand and a light-touch switch. This switch provided an auditory click for feedback. The switch was placed on the right side of his lap tray. This was frustrating for Eric, because he had to pick his hand up, move it over to the switch, and then place it down on the switch. Due to erratic arm movements, Eric had difficulty keeping his hand on the switch to activate the fan. A slanted surface with a cut-out recessed area for the switch was placed on his lap tray. Eric rested his forearm and hand on the slanted surface, and when he was ready to press the switch, he moved his hand toward the midline, his hand dropped into the recessed area on top of the switch, and the fan was activated. This arrangement made access easier for Eric than did placing the switch directly on the lap tray.

Eric's head movements were assessed next. The AT team wanted to compare his hand movement using the slanted surface with his ability to use the right side of his head for switch pressing. The Slim Armstrong mount from AbleNet was used to mount the switch. It was clamped to the back side support of his wheelchair so that the switch could be positioned by the right side of his head. The wobble switch was used first. This switch did not have an auditory click but was sensitive to movement from any direction; if it became slightly displaced, it could still be activated without difficulty. The occupational therapist on the AT team placed the wobble switch so that Eric could press it with the right temporal area of his head by laterally tilting his head. This movement did not elicit primitive reflexes and used a less abnormal path of motion and less force than did his hand movement. Additional information on head tilt is provided in Chapter 3.

Eric displayed some difficulty with the wobble switch. He could not tell when the side of his head was near it. He would press it accidentally and activate the fan before he was actually ready to do so. He unintentionally pressed the switch several times during the assessment. This situation may have been improved through changing the position of the switch, but Eric was becoming increasingly frustrated using it while trying to blow bubbles. Thus, the wobble switch proved to be too sensitive.

As an alternative, the lever switch from Zygo was chosen. The lever switch had a click that Eric could hear on activation. This feature was important because the switch would not be in his line of vision. The lever switch has a soft, spongy outer cover, which was replaced with an octopus soap holder to increase tactile feedback. This change of cover increased Eric's awareness of when the side of his head had made contact with the surface of the switch.

Eric displayed more control over the lever switch when compared with the wobble switch. In addition, Eric drooled less, exhibited fewer excess motions with his legs, and was more consistent in pressing the switch on command when using the lever switch.

Next, the therapist turned her attention to finding a permanent mounting system that would best suit Eric's needs. The therapist chose the Two-sided mounting system by Zygo, which uses rods that attach to both sides of the wheelchair back. This Two-sided mounting system provided stability as Eric pressed the switch. This mounting system attached to the back supports of Eric's wheelchair and did not interfere with other activities in which Eric was engaged throughout the day.

The final recommendation was for Eric to use a tilting motion with the right side of his head to activate the lever switch, with the octopus soap holder attached to it and the Two-sided mounting system. Although Eric needed some practice with this system, he began using it for academic tasks within a few weeks.

Case Study

RACHEL

Rachel was diagnosed with a C2–3 spinal cord injury 4 years ago as the result of an automobile accident. At the time, she was 18 years old, had recently graduated from high school, and had planned to go to college. Due to the spinal cord injury, she was quadriplegic and was ventilator dependent. She could not speak or move any part of her body except for facial muscles. Due to the tracheostomy, her ability to communicate was limited to mouthing words and facial expressions.

Rachel had been in and out of rehabilitation hospitals and was now coming to terms with her new lifestyle. She was beginning to take responsibility for her care and set some long-range goals. One of her goals was to start college on a part-time basis, majoring in communication arts. Her parents and the rehabilitation hospital staff supported her decision. The occupational therapist from the rehabilitation hospital knew of an occupational therapist who specialized in AT in a clinic in another facility. Rachel was referred there.

Rachel came to the assessment accompanied by her parents. At the time of the assessment, she was using a full recline Invacare wheelchair with a Jay cushion. A head roll was used to maintain her head in midline and to prevent neck hyperextension. At the time of the evaluation, Rachel was investigating the possibilities of driving a powered wheelchair. As a result of her treatment at the rehabilitation hospital, she had become adept at using a Sip and Puff Page Turner and a Sip and Puff to play Nintendo games.

Rachel's main reason for coming to the AT clinic was to explore methods that would allow her to complete homework assignments, tests, and term papers in college. Due to the control Rachel had of her facial muscles, she was shown switches that could be mounted near her face or around her head. All of these switches could be plugged into a personal computer and would allow operation of adaptive software. Rachel tried using the P-Switch (PRC), the infrared (Words+), and the tongue switch and body switch (both by APT Technology Inc., formerly known as Du-It Controls Systems Group). A tongue touch keypad (New-Abilities) switch would have been examined, but at the time of the assessment, it was still in experimental stages and was not available.

Rachel evaluated the effectiveness of each switch. One at a time, each switch was connected to a pleasant-sounding buzzer. As the therapist held the switch in place, Rachel activated it. Once Rachel had the "feel" of the switch, she was asked to press it on command and then either two or three times in rapid succession, depending on the therapist's direction. Pressing the switch on command helped Rachel and the therapist determine whether Rachel would be able to adequately use this switch for scanning or Morse code.

Rachel used each switch. Then, with the help of her mother to interpret, she stated her preferences for using each switch. The placement of the tongue switch bothered Rachel. Her chin and mouth would be hidden from others if the switch were mounted within her reach. She disliked the appearance this would present to others. Next, she used the body switch on the right side of her head near the back of her headrest. She could press the switch but could not consistently release it. In addition, the therapist felt that after traveling in the wheelchair, her position might be altered just enough for the switch to be out of reach; therefore, the body switch was ruled out. The P-Switch was secured to her forehead with an elastic band. Rachel was unable to demonstrate adequate control over this switch to warrant examination of mounting and activation options.

Following trial of the P-Switch, she used the Sip and Puff tube (pneumatic switch by PRC). Because of her experience in the rehabilitation hospital, she demonstrated adequate control of lip closure and sipping and puffing. She liked the control she had over the switch but was unhappy with the switch mounting because it covered part of her face. However, she preferred this switch to the tongue switch. It was smaller, covered less of her face, and she was able to reach it with her lips and remove it as needed.

The last switch that the therapist tried was the infrared switch by Words+. This switch is secured to eyeglass frames or a baseball cap. The infrared sensor is positioned so that it detects eye movement or an eye blink. Rachel could operate the switch on command, for a predetermined length of time, and send a series of eye blinks so that the switch activated in rapid succession. This appeared to be the switch over which Rachel had the most control and that she felt most comfortable using. She was not bothered by wearing eyeglasses, and if she chose, she could have the switch placed on a baseball cap occasionally for a change in position. Rachel also felt that this switch was the most cosmetically appealing.

In addition, because Rachel had experience using the Sip and Puff switch, it was recommended that this switch be purchased as well. This was done for two reasons. First, if the eyeglass frames became heavy and made her feel tired, she could substitute her switch control from the infrared switch to the Sip and Puff switch. This switch uses different facial muscles, giving the ones around her eye a rest. Also, a second switch provides another switch activation site from which Rachel can control her environment. Further, this Sip and Puff switch is really two switches, one for sip and one for puff, thereby opening up additional possibilities. As Rachel becomes accustomed to her equipment, she may find that additional switches give her more control and the ability to complete tasks more quickly. Purchasing a second switch now will give her more options later on as she becomes familiar with the equipment and begins to push it to its limits or purchase additional equipment.

Next, software programs were examined. Rachel was shown Morse code and scanning software programs. For evaluation purposes, she learned how to produce the letters "a" (short signal, long signal), "h" (three short signals), "o" (three long signals), "c" (long, short, long, short signal), and "d" (long, short, short signal). Rachel found Morse code difficult to use and made several errors. Using a scanning program, she learned within a few minutes the basic principles of indicating a letter and then a word and was writing short messages. She had immediate success with the scanning program and was enthusiastic about learning how to use it fully.

Because she did not have an augmentative communication system at the time of the evaluation, a scanning program that would allow her to speak and perform word-processing tasks was recommended. In this way, she would have the additional advantage of being able to prepare messages ahead of class, store them, and use them during class discussions. She would also be able to use the telephone, thus expanding communication opportunities with family and friends.

The following recommendations were made: the infrared and Sip and Puff switches; a computer with a hard disk large enough to hold the scanning, speech output, and word-processor software; MultiVoice voice synthesize (Words+); and a speakerphone.

STUDY QUESTIONS

1. Develop a switch hierarchy that will take an individual from initial introduction to a single switch to keyboard access. Keep in mind switch characteristics as well as the access features of a typical computer keyboard for which skills will need to be developed.
2. As indicated in this chapter, switches attached to toys are intended to be a means to an end for a child, and not an end in and of themselves. Thus, it is not enough to give a child a switch toy and revel in his or her ability to turn it on. We must then ask ourselves how to increase the complexity of the task, with the end result being giving the child more control over the environment. In applying this concept to an adult with both physical and cognitive limitations, to what might you attach a switch, and how could the complexity of the activity be increased?

REFERENCES

Bambara, L., Spiegel-McGill, P., Shores, R., & Fox, J. (1984). A comparison of reactive and nonreactive toys on severely handicapped children's manipulative play. *Journal of the Association for Persons with Severe Handicaps*, *9*, 142–149.

Goosens', C., & Crain, S. (1992). *Utilizing switch interfaces with children who are severely physically challenged*. Austin, TX: Pro-Ed.

Musselwhite, C.R. (1986). *Adaptive play for special needs children*. Boston: College-Hill Publication.

Scott-Taplin, C. (1988). Decisions, decisions—Narrowing the choices. *Communication Outlook*, *10*(2), 15–16.

Zygo Industries, Inc. (1995). Catalog, Tools of the Trade.

Companies That Sell Switches and Toys That Are Switch Ready

AbleNet Inc.
1081 Tenth Ave. S.E.
Minneapolis, MN 55414-1312
800-322-0956

APT Technology Inc. (formerly
  Du-It Controls Systems Group)
8765 Township Rd. No. 513
Shreve, OH 44676-9421
216-567-2001

Crestwood Company
6625 N. Sidney Place
Milwaukee, WI 53209-3259
414-352-5678

Don Johnston, Incorporated
PO Box 639
1000 N. Rand Rd.
Building 115
Wauconda, IL 60084-0639
800-999-4660

Tash
Unit 1-91 Station St.
Ajax, Ontario
Canada L1S 3H2
800-463-5685

Toys for Special Children
385 Warburton Ave.
Hastings-on-Hudson, NY 10706
914-478-0960

Words+, Inc.
400015 Sierra Highway
Building B-145
Palmdale, CA 93550
800-869-8521

Zygo Industries, Inc.
PO Box 1008A
Portland, OR 97207-1008
800-234-6006

APPENDIX B

Control Units for Electrical Appliances

Battery Device Adapter
PowerLink 2
Switch Latch and Timer
AbleNet Inc.
1081 Tenth Ave. S.E.
Minneapolis, MN 55414-1312
800-322-0956

Mounting Systems

Slim Armstrong
Universal Switch Mounting System
AbleNet Inc.
1081 Tenth Ave. S.E.
Minneapolis, MN 55414-1312
800-322-0956

Crestwood Company
Communication Aids for Children
    & Adults
6625 N. Sidney Place
Milwaukee, WI 53209
414-352-5678

Prentke-Romich Company
1022 Heyl Road
Wooster, OH 44691
800-262-1984

Toys for Special Children
385 Warburton Ave.
Hastings-on-Hudson, NY 10706
914-478-0960

Adaptive Fixtures Kit
One- and Two-Sided Mounting
    Systems
Zygo Industries, Inc.
PO Box 1008
Portland, OR 97207
800-234-6006

CHAPTER 5

LOW-TECHNOLOGY INTERFACE DEVICES

ASSESSMENT

OTHER FACTORS TO CONSIDER

LOW-TECHNOLOGY DEVICES
Placement of Keyboards and
   Communication Boards
Slanted Surface
Handheld Devices
Keyboard Adaptations
Keyguards

Physical Head Pointers
Stabilizer Methods
Suction-Cup Hand Holds

CASE STUDIES

APPENDIX: Handheld Devices and
   Technology Enhancers

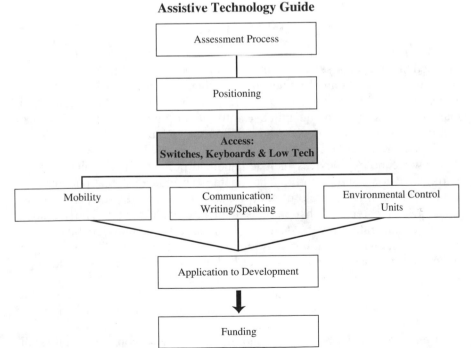

Assistive Technology Guide

Assessment Process

Positioning

**Access:
Switches, Keyboards & Low Tech**

Mobility | Communication:
Writing/Speaking | Environmental Control
Units

Application to Development

Funding

Providing high-technology devices alone can be insufficient to increase independence. Low-technology devices link the individual within the high-technology device. Low-technology devices enhance the potential of high technology to increase independence. Just like high-technology devices, low-technology devices must be evaluated for their appropriateness in a complete package to improve function. In this chapter, low-technology devices are discussed separately from access and input methods for the sake of clarity.

Here is an everyday example of how low technology and high technology work together. Short, able-bodied individuals have difficulty driving cars that have large plush driving seats. It is difficult for them to see over the steering wheel and reach the gas and brake pedals at the same time. With the seat in the most upright position and pulled as far forward as possible, they are able to drive the car (a high-technology device) without a low-technology device. However, they still strain to look out the windshield and to reach the pedals. Thus, they tire more quickly when driving this car than taller people. Two cushions, low-technology devices, one to sit on and one to place at their backs adjust the position enough so they do not strain to look out the windshield or to reach the pedals. They are more comfortable, more alert, and able to drive for longer periods before tiring when they use low-technology devices to assist them. Because of their modified seating, they may be better drivers.

The low-technology devices discussed in this chapter are primarily used in conjunction with computers, augmentative communication devices, and environmental control units.

ASSESSMENT

Optimally, the assessment for low-technology devices is completed in conjunction with the assessment for input methods. When the assessment for input methods is being conducted, the therapist may try several low-technology devices, using one or several of the assessments discussed in Chapter 3. This provides quantitative information about how the individual used the low-technology device and if it appears to have assisted the individual in using a particular input method.

Low-technology devices include handheld pointers, head pointers, keyboard adaptations, and so forth. When there is an indication that one or more of these devices may be helpful, they are shown to the individual adult, or to the child and parent. Each device is then briefly described. The therapist usually demonstrates how the device is used, because the individual may have no experience with it, and it may appear peculiar or odd. Then, using a keyboard or assessment board as described in Chapter 3, the low-technology devices are assessed. Once the individual has been given the opportunity to become familiar with each device, the therapist can introduce the Green Dot Test, or some other method of collecting qualitative and anecdotal information, and assess the usefulness of the device.

Regardless of the assessment chosen, it should be consistent across all devices so that information can be compared. In addition, the individual should indicate which device "feels" best to him or her. This is the one the individual feels the most comfortable wearing or using and the one with which the individual feels she or he has the most control. Based on this information, the therapist recommends equipment that best links the individual to his or her high-technology device(s).

At times the individual must use the device for a longer period than just during the assessment before a realistic recommendation can be made. Two or three device options can be field tested, each for an extended period (a day or a week). Information can be kept at the end of each hour or day regarding such factors as fatigue, ease of use, skin chafing, and accuracy. Assessments conducted over time provide information about device utility when the individual is in a variety of situations and has a range of energy levels. This method provides information that is difficult to gather when the entire assessment takes place in 1 day.

OTHER FACTORS TO CONSIDER

Other factors must be considered when choosing low technology to work with high-technology devices:

1. Can the individual independently don and doff the device?
    If the answer is no, can he or she be taught to independently don the device?
    If not, how will the individual be able to use the low-technology device when it is needed?
2. Whose job will it be to make sure that the individual has the device and help to put it on?
    Will it stay on all day?
    Will it be available on the wheelchair?
3. Are there other activities the individual engages in during the day with which the device will interfere? How will this issue be resolved?

The more the device fits in with the other activities, the better the chance that it will be used. In addition, the other people in the individual's daily routine need to be alerted to the intended purpose of the device, when it is to be used, and how to properly adjust the device to the individual. The individual also needs to be his or her own advocate. When possible, the individual needs to know when the device is to be used, how to instruct others regarding proper placement and adjustment, when it is to be taken off, and where it is to be stored to avoid losing it.

LOW-TECHNOLOGY DEVICES

Placement of Keyboards and Communication Boards

Although keyboards are not considered low-technology devices, the placement of keyboards can be considered a type of low technology. Placement of all equipment can be critical to the individual's ability to use the device. Placement can affect fatigue level, accuracy, and speed, and the keyboards should be positioned so they can be used efficiently. Individuals who use only one hand for typing may find it easier to use the keyboard on the same side as the preferred hand. In this way, the individual does not have to reach far to activate all keys. The individual can keep his or her arm close to the body, which may increase accuracy and reduce fatigue. In other situations, the keyboard may need to be at an angle on the opposite side of the body. Some individuals find it easier to keep the arm extended for efficient keyboard use. Keeping the keyboard perpendicular and at the midline to the body is not ideal for everyone.

Slanted Surface

A slanted surface, a surface providing forearm support, can be used with single switches, keyboards, or communication boards (Fig. 5–1). Some individuals find key pressing (with fingers or a head pointer) easier when the keyboard is slanted rather than flat on the table. A slanted surface elevates the keyboard slightly and provides forearm support, which may help increase accuracy, prevent fatigue, and decrease extraneous movements. It can also be used in combination with a keyguard. The individual rests his or her forearm on the slanted surface and the hand on the keyguard or wrist rest. When assessing the use of a slanted surface, a 1-, 2-, and 3-inch three-ring notebook can be used for assessment. For permanent use, a slanted surface should be fabricated from a sturdy material. They keyboard can be mounted to the slanted surface with a nonslip type of material or Poly-Loc.

Handheld Devices

At times, high-technology devices, such as keyboards connected to computers, are not sufficient by themselves to provide communicating, writing access, and so forth. Handheld devices are generally used to improve the individual's ability to operate keyboards, augmentative communication devices, communication boards, and environmental control units. When the individual appears to have enough upper extremity control to use a keyboard but insufficient control over one or more movements, handheld devices can be introduced during the access assessment. The purpose of handheld devices is to improve pointing ability. This eliminates the need to point with an extended finger while locating the desired key or item on a communication board.

Examples of handheld devices that assist in pointing include the following:

1. Dolphin Pointer
2. Keyguard Slider
3. Universal Cuff
4. Built-up pencil or dowel

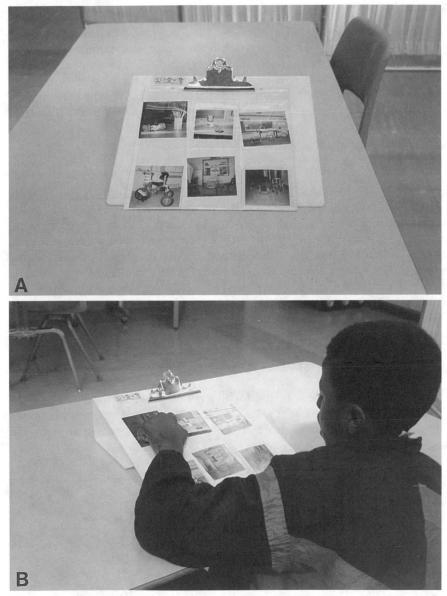

Figure 5–1. Slanted surface with communication board (*A*). Child using communication board with slanted surface (*B*).

5. Mouse adaptations
6. T-bar
7. Wanchik's Writer
8. Typing splints

Dolphin Pointer

This pointer, developed at the TRACE Center in Madison, Wisconsin (see Appendix), and named for its dolphin-like shape, assists individuals with pointing to items on a communication board (Fig. 5–2). The tip of the pointer is red to define the area that is the actual "pointer." This pointer works well for individuals who have cerebral palsy and excess movements. Instead of trying to use one finger as a pointer, the individuals hold on to the handle of the Dolphin Pointer and place the red tip over the desired item. The pointer and handle are sized for small hands.

Keyguard Slider

The Keyguard Slider (Fig. 5–3) is a modification of the Dolphin Pointer (from TRACE Center in Madison, Wisconsin) and is usually used in combination with a keyguard (see Appendix). The pointer component has been changed to a dowel that is positioned vertically. A wedge is adhered to the bottom surface of the pointer. The pointer rests on top of the keyguard. The individual moves the pointer over the keyguard, using a motion much like the one used when ironing. When the desired letter is under the tip of the dowel (pointer), the individual tips the pointer, inserting it into the hole in the keyguard, and the desired key is pressed.

Universal Cuff

The Universal Cuff can be used with a pencil or dowel placed in it (Figs. 5–4 and 5–5). When used with a keyguard, the individual can rest his or her hand directly over the keyboard and press the desired key. When using the

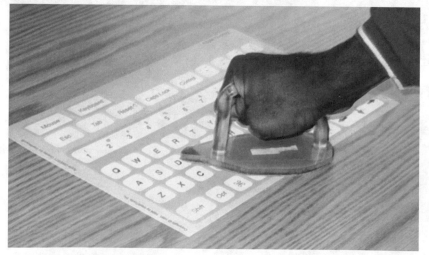

Figure 5–2. Dolphin-shaped pointer.

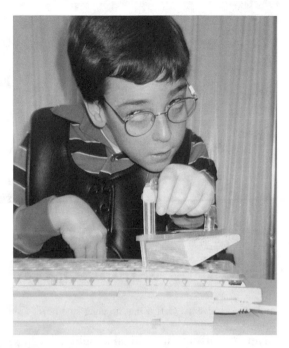

Figure 5–3. Keyguard Slider.

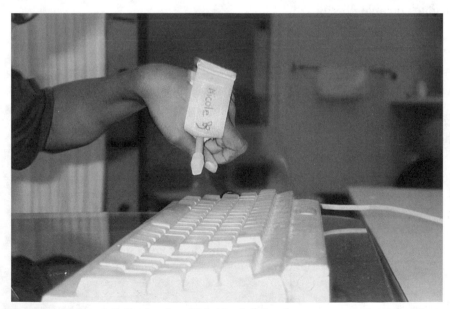

Figure 5–4. Universal Cuff using the radial side of the hand.

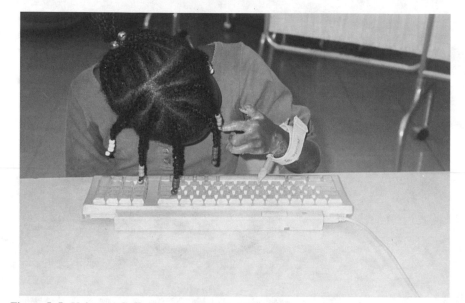

Figure 5–5. Universal Cuff using the ulnar side of the hand.

Universal Cuff, the individual should try it in several configurations, with the pencil on the radial side of the wrist between the thumb and index finger, and on the ulnar side of the hand with the pencil extending from the little finger. There is great variability in the best use of the device, and therefore much experimentation is needed to find the position in which the individual demonstrates optimal control.

Built-Up Pencil or Dowel

Pencils and dowels are built up in many ways. They can then be used to press the keys on a keyboard or other device. Examples include a built-up pencil holder, triangular pencil grips, molded pencil grips, foam tubing, and pencils inserted through Wiffle or rubber balls to increase grip surface area. The diameter of the ball depends on the size of the individual's hand.

Mouse Adaptations

Several software programs for personal computers (PCs) and Macintosh computers use a mouse and the keyboard for input methods. For some children, using the mouse requires more motor control than they have. There are several alternatives to using the mouse, including learning the keyboard alternatives, modifying the mouse, and using a track ball. The keyboard alternatives and a mouse modification are discussed here. The assessment for mice and track balls is discussed in Chapter 3.

A low-technology solution to the difficulty of performing computer commands when using the mouse is attaching Velcro to a strap that is placed around the individual's hand. The other piece of Velcro is attached to the palm rest on the mouse. When the individual places his or her hand on top of the mouse, the mouse sticks to the Velcro that is attached to the hand. This stabilizes the mouse to the hand and allows the individual to drag the mouse without having to hold onto it. It allows the individual to concentrate on dragging the mouse to move the cursor to the desired location on the screen and then clicking the mouse button as needed to perform an action. This option is particularly useful for drawing programs that rely on mouse use extensively. When the mouse is not required, the individual keeps the strap on the hand and peels off the Velcro, just like releasing any other device with Velcro attachments. The individual can still use the keyboard with the Velcro strap in place on the hand.

T-Bar

A T-bar is made from two dowels that are attached to form a "T" shape (Fig. 5–6). The individual grasps the bar with the pointer extended between the middle and ring fingers. The individual then uses the T-bar to press keys on the keyboard or augmentative communication device or to indicate items on a communication board. For individuals who have difficulty maintaining a grasp, Velcro can be used for a hand strap and fastened to the T-bar. The

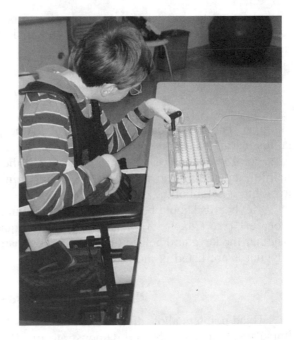

Figure 5–6. T-bar.

T-bar is used with or without a keyguard and works well with many keyboards.

Wanchik's Writer

These splints provide wrist and index finger support. They are appropriate to try for individuals who have spinal cord injuries or disabilities and need additional support to use the index finger as a pointer. The wrist support is also useful if the individual's wrist has a tendency to flex. Depending on the individual's control over the right and left hands, one or two splints may be recommended. They are sold by Be OK! (see Appendix).

Typing Splints

Slip-On Typing/Keyboard Aids can be tried when the individual has adequate wrist control but limited finger control. These aids replace the index finger in a one-finger typing action. One or two splints are used, depending on the individual's ability. They are sold by Be OK! (see Appendix).

This list of interface devices is not exhaustive. It provides additional ideas to assist therapists in problem solving with their clients regarding accessing high-technology devices.

Keyboard Adaptations

Adapted keyboards enable people to use computer keyboards, augmentative communication keyboards, environmental control unit keyboards, and so forth.

Keyguards

Keyguards (Fig. 5–7) are usually made of clear plastic material and fit snugly over the keyboard. Holes are cut in the plastic to allow a finger or stylus instrument to press one key at a time. Keyguards eliminate the pressing of several keys at once when trying to reach the desired key. They are also helpful in guiding the finger or dowel instrument to the desired key and avoiding a neighboring key.

Keyboards should be tested with and without keyguards using the Green Dot Test (see Chapter 3). This test provides quantitative information as to whether the keyguard helped or hindered keyboard entry. Companies that sell keyguards are listed in the Appendix.

Physical Head Pointers

Head pointers allow direct-selection access for people with severe motor impairment. Individuals who demonstrate insufficient hand motion use them

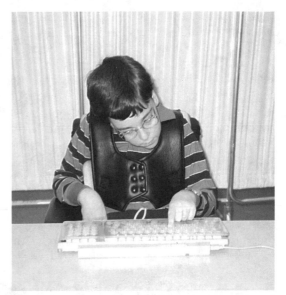

Figure 5–7. Keyguard.

to access switches or keyboards. Head pointers fasten to the head and must be adjusted to fit. The pointer comes over the head, around the face, or under the chin. If they are loose, they are difficult to use because the pointer will move as the individual applies force.

Individuals may not be accustomed to using their head as a method of pointing and indicating choices. The therapist and the individual should not become discouraged if the first few attempts to use the head pointer are not successful. It may take several practice or training sessions before the individual becomes proficient at using the head pointer. A slanted surface can be used to place the keyboard at an angle. This may provide easier access when using a physical head pointer.

Involving children in play activities using the head pointer can help teach head-pointing skills. For adults, exercises using the head pointer would be appropriate. At the onset of head-pointing training, it is advisable to avoid keyboards or other devices with small target areas. Using small targets for practice may be frustrating and make a negative impression on the individual. Larger targets are better at the beginning of training. For children, the head pointer can be replaced with other tools to allow the child to paint, draw, and knock down towers. Activities that can be used during music time are playing the drum, triangle, and other rhythm instruments. Other musical activities that may require more coordination are playing a xylophone or toy piano. These keys are larger than the keyboard keys, yet they take more precision to press than do free-form drawing and painting activities. Games, such as checkers, large concentration game boards, or memory games, are also suitable activities. Computer games using alternate keyboards programmed for larger keys also work for practicing head-pointing skills. For adults, drawing, painting, playing games, and practicing with increasingly smaller targets are suitable. Once some initial success has been achieved, the activities can be more keyboard directed, such as using computer games.

Some individuals or their families will reject physical head pointers because of their appearance. Disguising a head pointer may make it more appealing to the individual, although some feel that this is deceptive. If "camouflaging" appears appropriate, find out the individual's interests. Head gear that complements that interest can be made or purchased. For example, if the individual has a favorite baseball team, a baseball cap with the insignia of that team can be placed on top of the pointer. This allows the head pointer to take on new significance and makes it less obvious. An example for young girls is to pretend it is the headdress of a ballerina; the head pointer can be decorated with ribbons, feathers, and glitter to take on the appearance of a tiara, something that a ballerina might wear for a performance. A list of companies that sell head pointers is provided in the Appendix.

Stabilizer Methods

Some low-technology devices are used to stabilize limbs. Usually, the nondominant arm or both arms are stabilized in some fashion. Generally, stabilizing the nondominant arm or hand improves control over the trunk, and therefore over the dominant arm or hand. It gives the nondominant arm or hand a place to stabilize while increasing the base of support. When the head is being used to activate the high-technology device, both arms or hands may need to be stabilized. Stabilizing also prevents the nondominant arm from excess movement, adding to an overall stability.

Suction-Cup Hand Holds

Suction-cup hand holds provide a handle for the individual to use with the nondominant hand (Figs. 5–8 and 5–9). They come in vertical and horizontal models. The one the individual uses depends on whether he or she has a better grasp when the wrist is neutral or prone. The dowel is available for the individual to grasp with the nondominant hand while he or she uses the dominant hand to operate a keyboard or other input device. He or she releases the dowel when the task is completed. Using this low-technology equipment provides freedom of movement and does not confine the arm. It is permanently affixed to the lap tray or table through the suction cups on the bottom of the dowel rods. Once the dowel is positioned, it generally does not need to be moved and is maintenance free. However, it may occupy space on the lap tray that is needed for other activities, such as the communication board or lunch tray. The suction-cup hand holds can be purchased from Rifton (see Appendix).

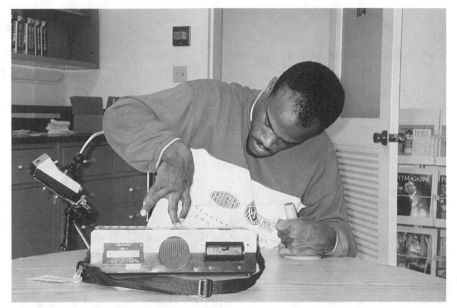

Figure 5–8. Suction-cup hand hold—vertical.

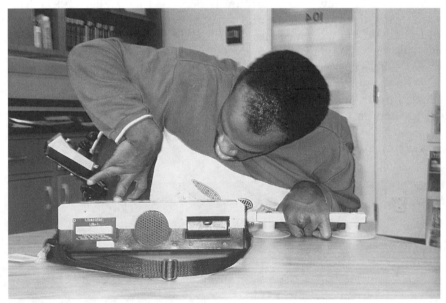

Figure 5–9. Suction-cup hand hold—horizontal.

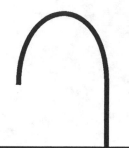

Figure 5–10. Hook with lap tray.

The Hook

The hook looks like the curved part of a shepherd's hook or the curved part of a wooden cane and is described by Goosens' & Crain (1992) (Fig. 5–10). It provides support similar to that of the dowels. The individual is able to use and remove his or her arm independently. The major difference is that there is no grasping required. The individual slips his or her arm under the device. The hook part of the device holds the arm in place while the individual accesses a switch or keyboard. It is usually covered with a soft material to avoid skin abrasions. It attaches to the lap tray with screws.

Lap Tray

Another method to increase hand or head control is to place the arm(s) underneath the lap tray. This procedure is described by Trefler (1982). The experiences of three individuals with athetoid cerebral palsy using lap trays to restrain their arm movement are described. Each individual accomplished an activity (direct a light sensor, press a chin switch to operate a self-feeder, or use an E-Tran eye-gaze communication system) with more speed or ability than when the arms were not restrained. Another study of lap tray use was conducted by Trefler, Monahan, and Nwaobi (1986) using 14 subjects. This study focused on family attitudes regarding tray use. Generally, families of people using the lap tray restraint were pleased with the outcomes. Further, the trays increased function for the subjects.

Case Study

AMY

Amy is 12 years old and has cerebral palsy. The purpose of the evaluation by the assistive technology (AT) team was to improve her ability to use her communication board. The communication board has the alphabet printed in the middle in 1-inch squares and words printed on the periphery of the board. At this time, she is not a candidate for a high-technology device. She uses her board throughout the day in her special classroom. She spends half a day in a program to help her transition into a workshop setting. She is learning to operate a switch connected to a machine that seals plastic bags once hardware nails have been dropped into them.

Her hand movements are erratic, and it is difficult for others to know which letter or words she is pointing to on her communication board. She uses her index finger to point to items on her communication board. She has difficulty extending her index finger while pointing to the desired letter or word, due to excess movements. Thus, much guessing is involved in Amy's communication.

Amy's communication board is flat on her lap tray. When she points, she usually abducts her arm and does not rest her forearm on the lap tray. This puts her in an unsteady position for using her index finger as a pointer. To try to increase stability and improve accuracy, the communication board was placed on a slanted surface to encourage Amy to rest her forearm. Nevertheless, Amy continued abducting her arm when using her communication board and required constant verbal cuing to lower her arm. This was frustrating for Amy, so the slanted surface was discarded.

The next item that was tried was the Dolphin Pointer. The Dolphin Pointer increased Amy's accuracy while pointing to the desired item; however, she had great difficulty maintaining a grasp on the handle. Her fingers involuntarily released the pointer. It became clear to the AT team that the Dolphin Pointer would have to be attached to her hand so that she did not have to grasp and point with it simultaneously. A modified Dolphin Pointer was made for her. Lexan plastic was cut as if forming the base for the Dolphin Pointer. Velcro was attached to the top surface. Velcro and fabric were sewed together to resemble a watchband. The Velcro watchband was placed around Amy's wrist. Amy placed her wrist, with the watchband around it, on the velcro attached to the modified Dolphin Pointer. With this pointing device, she rested her forearm on the communication board voluntarily and used an ironing motion to move the pointer across the communication board. She needed to concentrate on moving the pointer to the appropriate letter or word but no longer needed to maintain an extended index finger. Her ability to use her communication board effectively improved. Communication partners were more certain about which letter or word she was pointing to, and it took less time for Amy to complete messages.

Amy was not able to don the modified pointer independently. Her teacher in her classroom assumed the responsibility of putting the pointer on in the morning, taking it off and placing it in Amy's backpack during lunch, replacing it on her hand for the afternoon, and placing it in her backpack at the end of the day. With this simple solution, Amy was able to communicate faster and more reliably. Others to whom she talked regularly were pleased with the improvement. It was easier to carry on a conversation with her because less guessing was involved.

Case Study

LARRY

Larry is a 21-year-old man with spastic cerebral palsy. He was referred to the AT clinic for an assessment concerning his workstation. He uses a powered wheelchair, has limited use of his arms and hands, and has adequate head control to consider using a head pointer. He has just accepted a position working at the local independent living center. However, he must be able to use a computer, perform some word processing, use a bulletin board system to download files, leave messages and post notices, use the telephone, and attend meetings. He referred himself to the AT clinic primarily to help him locate a telephone system that he could operate independently. The AT team also wanted to explore more efficient computer access methods.

Larry used a standard keyboard by typing with his nose. The keyboard is placed on a standard desk with no adaptations. He complained of neck and shoulder pain from using this position. In addition, he is unable to see what he is typing on the screen and he cannot execute commands that require keys to be pressed simultaneously. For telephone access, someone must dial and hold the receiver for him.

The first idea the AT team had was to have Larry try various head pointers. Zygo makes one that has sticks of various lengths and can be angled for easier use. The team also wanted to raise the keyboard slightly, using a slanted surface so Larry would not have to use as much neck flexion to type. Larry humored the team and tried the head pointer. However, he made it very clear to the team that he was not interested in using it. A head pointer was something else that he would have to either take time to put on himself or ask for help to put on. In addition, it was one more item to keep track of during the day. Therefore, head pointers were not an option. The team then decided to increase the angle of the slanted surface. A specialized holder was made for the keyboard so it was nearly vertical, and the computer screen was above it. Larry tried this keyboard holder. He found it acceptable. He could continue typing with his nose. Once it was in place in front of the monitor, nothing else was needed to use it. Larry was pleased with this setup.

He could see the computer screen to observe his work as he typed, and the neck pain was diminishing.

The next problem the team addressed was the telephone system. Larry evaluated a gooseneck receiver mount that held the handset with a simple mechanism that held down or released the dial tone button. His phone numbers could be stored in his computer, and the computer could be connected so that it would dial the telephone. This allowed Larry to have private conversations and not be hampered by wearing a head set. Larry found this system acceptable.

Larry has now been at this job for more than 1 year. His annual review by his employer was very positive. The interface devices have helped Larry perform his job. He no longer suffers chronic neck pain.

STUDY QUESTIONS

1. Low-technology adaptations for infants and toddlers may include items in addition to those described in this chapter. Consider how you might use such items as dycem or other nonslip material, Velcro pieces or straps, plastic links, bias tape with snaps to augment a small child's ability to access a switch attached to a toy, or the toy itself.
2. How might you adapt something like a suction-cup hand hold to make it more appealing to a 13-year-old child? An adult?

REFERENCES

Goosens', C., & Crain, S. (1992). Utilizing switch interfaces with children who are severely physically impaired. Austin, TX: Pro-Ed.

Trefler, E., Monahan, L., & Nwaobi, O. M. (1986). Functional arm restraint for children with athetoid cerebral palsy (pp. 60–61). Minneapolis: RESNA 9th Annual Conference.

Trefler, E. (1982). Arm restraints during functional activities. *American Journal of Occupational Therapy*, *36* (9), 599–600.

Handheld Devices and Technology Enhancers

Dolphin Pointer and Keyguard
Slider
TRACE Research and Development
Center
Waisman Center
1500 Highland Ave.
Madison, WI 53705-2280
608-262-6966

Headpointers
Zygo Industries, Inc.
PO Box 1008A
Portland, OR 97207-1008
800-234-6006

Keyguards
Don Johnston, Incorporated
PO Box 639
1000 N. Rand Rd.
Building 15
Wauconda, IL 60084-0639

Keyguards, Wanchik's Writer,
Slip-On Typing/Keyboard Aid,
Headpointers
Be OK! Fred Sammons Inc.
PO Box 32
Brookfield, IL 60513
800-323-5547

Suction-Cup Hand Holds
Rifton
PO Box 901
Rifton, NY 12471-0901
800-374-3866

POWERED AND MANUAL WHEELCHAIR MOBILITY

Susan Johnson Taylor, OTR, and David Kreutz, PT

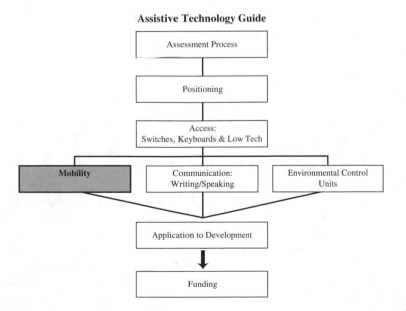

Assistive Technology Guide

FACTORS AFFECTING THE DECISION
BETWEEN POWERED AND
MANUAL MOBILITY

When evaluating clients for mobility, the therapist must first ask whether the client will use powered mobility, manual mobility, or both. A precise formula for deciding between a powered and a manual wheelchair would help in the decision process; however, as with most problems that involve interfacing human beings with technology, there is no black-and-white matrix to guide consumers, clinicians, and suppliers toward an easy solution.

It may be useful to talk about what mobility is or should be. The goal of mobility is to get from point "A" to point "B." People without physical limitations that hinder mobility move freely within their environments without giving it much thought. Once a physical limitation is imposed, movement becomes compromised and difficult. The goal becomes moving between points in the most efficient manner possible and still having energy to function once they get there. Some therapists are reluctant to provide consumers with the most efficient mobility, preferring them to use every bit of their physical skill to continue walking. These therapists fear they will encourage laziness and dependence if they suggest an alternate method of mobility. However, most people without physical disabilities do not walk around with weights around each leg to make sure they do not become too lazy.

Consumers must be armed with the facts before they can decide what form of mobility suits them best (Taylor & Kreutz, 1994). Many factors affect the decision to use powered or manual mobility. Ideally, the consumer, clinician, and rehabilitation technology supplier come together to reach this decision.

Some basic areas to evaluate are similar to a seating evaluation: functional status, cognitive status, vision, and environmental or transportation considerations.

Functional Status

Some types of injuries and conditions do not allow the client to propel a manual wheelchair. Generally, the therapist is looking at strength, range of motion (as discussed in Chapter 2), the effects of abnormal tone and reflexes on the ability to propel, and related medical conditions. For example, a client with a C-4 spinal cord injury or severe cerebral palsy would not be able to propel a wheelchair; therefore, the therapist would evaluate that person's ability to control a powered wheelchair if independent mobility was the client's goal. However, many individuals could physically use either, such as a person with a C6–7 spinal cord injury or mild cerebral palsy. A client may choose to use a manual wheelchair even if it is not the most efficient form of mobility for him or her. However, when a client is propelling a manual wheelchair without fully functional upper extremities, it is the therapist's responsibility to educate the client about the known and suspected long-term physical effects of propelling the wheelchair (Pentland, 1992). For some clients, having access to both powered and manual mobility is ideal. For example, a student with enough strength and coordination to propel short distances, such as in the home, may want a powered wheelchair for moving around the college campus or for other long distances.

Another important factor is whether the client can independently relieve pressure and shift his or her weight. A client who has no ability to move independently may require a powered tilt or recline unit. To be independent in mobility, a powered tilt or recline must be mounted on a powered wheelchair. It would be too heavy to push if mounted on a manual wheelchair base.

If a client elicits abnormal tone or reflexes while propelling a manual wheelchair, causing deforming postures, it may be necessary to consider a powered wheelchair to avoid long-term orthopedic and postural problems. The client may have conditions such as chronic obstructive pulmonary disease or a heart condition that prevents him or her from exerting as much energy as is needed for propulsion. Individuals with a progressive disorder, such as multiple sclerosis, may have difficulty with fatigue and, although physically capable of propelling the wheelchair, may not have the endurance.

Cognitive Status

This area is divided into two categories: (1) clients with cognitive impairments secondary to a head injury, developmental delay, or other factors, and (2) children. When a client is cognitively impaired, the therapist must be aware of several areas, including memory, problem-solving abilities, and impulse control. The therapist can combine that information with knowledge of the client's motor planning and perceptual-motor abilities. With that information, the therapist can structure the evaluation and know what to look for in terms of responses from the client. Some information can be gathered ahead of time from standard occupational therapy, physical therapy, speech pathology, and psychological evaluations. Unless it is obvious that the client cannot use a powered or manual wheelchair, the therapist should complete the evaluation and have the client try the equipment. Many clients are able to use compensatory strategies to adapt to some of these difficulties.

Children as young as 18 months are capable of understanding and using powered mobility. However, mobility for these children must be treated just like that for any other child; young children require supervision until they are old enough to handle the mobility safely and independently (Butler, 1988). Independent mobility is essential for children and should be allowed whenever possible, because by exploring and testing their environments, children learn perceptual-motor and social skills (Butler, 1991). Within the last 10 to 15 years, clinicians and researchers have begun to study the effects of the provision of early mobility, particularly powered mobility. In a Seattle study, children as young as 24 months were able to operate powered devices with supervision (Butler, Okamoto & McKay, 1983). A Swedish study found that children trained with powered-mobility devices became less dependent on complete verbal control of their environments. In addition, not only did these children maintain interest in their therapy goals, but they became more willing to participate (Paulsson & Christofferson, 1984). They were found overall to be much more interactive with peers and to initiate these interactions rather than waiting for other children to approach them. They began to view themselves as competent human beings.

The arguments from therapists, parents, and teachers against providing early powered mobility revolve around several concerns: The children are too immature to be aware of safety issues with a powered device; the equipment is very expensive; and the children may lose interest in working toward therapy goals, such as walking. "Augmentative mobility" has become an approach for children who are nonambulatory or partially ambulatory (Butler, 1991). This means that efficient mobility does not have to be an all-or-nothing approach; it can be incorporated into an overall plan for the child. A child can be provided with the forms of mobility appropriate for the activity in which he or she is involved. For example, for getting around the school and outdoor play, a powered wheelchair may be preferred over crutches and braces.

Finally, inefficient ambulation can have deleterious physical effects that lead to poor school performance. In another study, children who were required to ambulate (children with braces and crutches or walkers) were found to exceed 60% to 70% of their maximal heart rate by the time they arrived in their classroom. This caused a statistically significant decrease in visual and motor performance, which had a negative impact on their academic performance (Butler, 1991).

Vision

Some visual testing, such as for acuity and visual-perceptual skills, can occur prior to the powered mobility evaluation. This testing provides the therapist with a baseline of the client's visual status. The true nature of most visual problems may not become apparent until the client actually tries the new methods of powered or manual mobility. Even a client with severe visual deficits may be able to negotiate familiar environments. On the other hand, powered mobility may not be advisable if a client is unable to discern dangerous situations. This may be true for patients with acuity problems and perceptual problems, such as unilateral neglect.

Transportation and Accessibility

The mode of transportation available to the client is discussed at the evaluation. The powered or manual wheelchair the client will be using must be measured. If the client already has a wheelchair and wants a new one, the therapist and rehabilitation technology supplier (RTS) should ask the client to show how the chair currently fits into his or her vehicle. This includes how the client or caregiver transfers and transports the powered or manual wheelchair. If the client drives from the chair, the relationship of the driving controls to the present chair and to the client's positioning within the chair should be examined.

Important measurements to ensure that the client will continue to fit into the existing vehicle and environments (e.g., home, school, work) include the overall width and length of the chair, the height of the client in the chair from the floor to the top of the head (for fitting into van door openings and inside the van), and the amount of clearance under the footrests (if the client drives from the chair and needs to drive over the lock-down). If this is a first wheelchair, contact the company that will be modifying the van so the chair and van will be compatible.

Accessibility issues also include the type of environment in which the client lives and how he or she plans to use the chair. For example, some clients use the chair almost as an off-road vehicle for going to town or over broken sidewalks, whereas others will use it primarily indoors. If possible, the therapist can make home visits to look at accessibility. Information about door widths, ramp access, turning spaces, and so forth can be collected from the client's home. Sometimes the RTS can take a trial wheelchair to the client's home, school, or office to ensure it will be functional.

Children using school transportation will need to have their school district's requirements reviewed prior to final prescription. Some do not accept certain types of wheelchairs or powered wheelchair batteries.

POWERED MOBILITY TECHNOLOGY AND EVALUATION

Powered Mobility Technology

A decade or so ago, powered mobility options were simple: A consumer could use either a microswitch or a proportional controller, which allowed little adjustment for individual physical skills. For individuals with high-technology needs, the solutions either were not available or were custom solutions, which were very expensive. With the advent of microcomputers, manufacturers were able to offer options for fine-tuning the electronics to correspond with physical need (Taylor, 1995).

Powered mobility technology varies with each manufacturer and chair; however, many features can be discussed in generic terms. As previously discussed, determining the type of powered wheelchair the client requires depends on the client's physical, functional, and environmental needs. A careful match of the type of chair and electronics results in a functional and cost-effective powered chair. The following sections define and discuss the parts of the powered wheelchair and how they function.

Controllers or Modules

The *controller* or *module* is the "brain" of the chair. It allows various performance parameters of the chair to be set for each client to suit individual physical and functional needs. Most modules are microprocessor controlled, which allows the information to be changed and saved as it would be on a computer. It also allows peripheral devices to be used. The controller allows certain types of inputs to be used and certain characteristics of these inputs to be modified according to changes in the client's functional needs. The following are some basic controller functions.

Proportional Versus Microswitch or Digital

The *input device* is the method by which the client operates the chair. Input devices are of two types: proportional or microswitch. A *proportional control* works like a gas pedal in a car: Speed is proportional to how hard the gas pedal is pushed. A standard joystick is proportional. If it is just barely pushed, the chair will go slowly. If pushed to its limits, the chair will go faster. A proportional control allows more fine maneuvering, particularly in tight spaces. A *microswitch,* or *digital, control* works more like a light switch; it is either on or off. When contacted or activated, it runs the chair at a constant speed until the pressure is removed.

Momentary Versus Latched

A *momentary control* operates only when the input device is being contacted. For example, as soon as the client removes his or her hand from the joystick, the chair stops. With a *latched control,* the input device is contacted once (such as a single hard puff on a Sip and Puff system), after which the chair continues forward until given the command to stop (in the case of a Sip and Puff system, a hard sip). Two directions, such as forward and reverse, can be operated in a latched mode (as described previously), while the left and right directions are operated in a momentary mode. The client would give a single hard puff and drive forward in a latched mode. Changes in course direction to the left or right would be provided in a momentary mode with soft sips and puffs.

Acceleration

Acceleration refers to how quickly the wheelchair reaches the top end of the speed from the starting point. Fast acceleration would provide an active user with a very responsive chair. Slow acceleration would allow a slow start for someone who has a difficult time adjusting to changes in speed and direction.

Deceleration or Braking

Deceleration, sometimes called braking, refers to how quickly the chair comes to a stop once input to the input device is discontinued. Fast deceleration tends to "throw" the person forward slightly. For a person with poor head or trunk control, this may not be desirable; he or she may need to come to a slower stop. On the other hand, if someone needs to come to a quick stop because of obstacles in his or her environment, a chair with quick reaction may be required.

Tremor Dampening

Tremor dampening tells the controller to ignore erratic input from the input device. This works only with proportional systems. For example, if a client had tremors of the upper extremity, tremor dampening would be engaged and adjusted so the client had a relatively straight course, despite the fact that he or she was unable to maintain fine control of the hand, upper extremity, or whatever body part was being used to control the input device.

High Speed, Low Speed, Turn Speed, and Forward-Reverse Ratio

These adjustments provide clients with the speed in each direction that best suits their needs. Each can be adjusted from 100%, which would be the fastest for each direction, down to a comfortable level for the client. Some chairs offer two programs — one setting for a slower, more manageable setting, such as indoors, and another for higher performance, such as outdoors. It is important to program these speeds for the types of environments within which they will be functioning. Tuning the wheelchair down too much on a surface such as a carpet could result in the wheelchair being unable to overcome the inertia of the wheels turning, particularly on sharp turns.

Short Throw

The *short-throw adjustment* is used with proportional controls. This decreases the range of motion of the input device (such as a joystick) necessary to activate the control. This is useful for clients who have decreased active (strength) or passive range of motion of the body part they are using for operating the input control.

Capability of Using Recline or Tilt Systems and Other Electronic Devices

Sometimes a client who has limited physical abilities will use one input control for a variety of functions, such as driving, operating a recline or tilt unit, and operating an environmental control unit or augmentative communication device. Each function has a separate circuit board in the controller that can be accessed through the input device. The client has a visual display that shows what "channel" or function is being used. By giving input through the input device, the client can change the function. For example, a client using a Sip and Puff straw as the input control could change from the drive function to the recline or tilt function and then to the environmental control function, all with the same Sip and Puff straw. A system that includes options for control of two or more functions through one input device is called an *integrated control* (Caves, 1994). An advantage of this type of control is that the user needs only one input method to access many functions. A disadvantage is that if one part of the system goes down, the user may lose all of the functions if there are not alternate inputs. Another disadvantage is that if the user is capable of using more than one input, this system can actually be slower because the user must input "channel changes" and wait for a response.

Reset Time

Reset time is used when the previous system is being used. It is the amount of time required for the wheelchair to enter stand-by mode, which can be likened to "neutral" mode in a car. If the client does not want the system to automatically go into reset, this feature can be turned off, and the client can initiate going into reset at will.

Wheelchair Bases

Wheelchair bases are available in many sizes and configurations and offer a variety of choices of electronics. Which base to use depends on the functional features the client requires. Powered wheelchair bases are either belt driven or direct drive. With a *belt-driven* system, the motor turns the pulleys on each side of the wheelchair, which turns the wheels. This method of operating a powered chair has been used for many years successfully. With time, the belts loosen, causing the wheelchair to react more slowly. Some of the pulley designs have a tendency to slip, especially during wet conditions. One design that works well are the belts with deep grooves, which make the chair less likely to slip. A *direct-drive* system has the motor connected directly to the wheels. This is a much more efficient system and makes for a more responsive chair, particularly outdoors. However, care must be taken to collect repair information from the RTS regarding which parts of chairs are likely to break down and who will perform repairs and maintenance.

Powered wheelchairs are broken down into the following categories: traditional powered wheelchairs, powered bases, high-performance powered wheelchairs, transportable powered wheelchairs, and add-on power packs. Scooters, although considered powered devices and not powered wheelchairs, are also discussed.

Traditional powered chairs have a large (20-inch) wheel in the rear with smaller (8- or 9-inch) casters in the front. For the most part, they are belt-driven wheelchairs. They perform well outdoors over relatively level surfaces and perform very well indoors. The electronics on these wheelchairs vary widely, from little adjustment to multifunction adjustments. The price rises according to the amount of adjustment available. Not unlike buying a car (some powered wheelchairs in many of these categories rival the prices of small cars), the key to buying this or any powered wheelchair is to buy into the electronics package the user needs. Keep in mind with the purchase of any of the wheelchairs that if the client who is being evaluated has a progressive or changing condition, the expense of flexible electronics up front may be worth the cost. Prices of wheelchairs can vary by thousands of dollars and can mean the difference between a model that has basic speed control to one that is highly adjustable.

With a *powered base,* the powered section is a separate unit from the seating unit. This allows a variety of seating units to be attached to the top of the base because the back post uprights are not an integral part of the structure of the chair. For example, a powered recline or tilt unit would attach directly to the top of the base. However, some of the seating units attach to a powered base with a single post, which may provide the users with a rocking motion as they travel over uneven surfaces. This can be particularly troubling for those whose tone or reflexes are induced by these types of sudden motions. In addition, because of the large balloon tires, they can be difficult for a caregiver to push when out of gear.

All powered bases have direct-drive motors. They tend to be heavy duty and will perform particularly well outdoors, including over challenging surfaces, such as areas of hilly grass and gravel, and will not sink as easily into soft surfaces, such as loose soil. Performance indoors may prove to be rough, especially on carpeted areas. They usually have large, wide front and rear wheels that provide a great deal of friction. Some (although not many) powered bases have the larger (15-inch) wheel in front with the caster in the rear. The Permobil wheelchair, shown in Figure 6–1, is one such chair. This wheelchair provides a superior turning radius, because the user is turning around his or her own body's pivot point. In addition, if the user has tight hamstrings that necessitate positioning the knees at 90 degrees or greater, this can be accommodated without worrying about the feet getting caught in the casters.

If the user already has a tie-down system, it needs to be checked carefully, because powered-base wheelchairs tie down differently than do traditional wheelchairs. This is especially an issue for a wheelchair with casters in the rear.

High-performance powered wheelchairs represent a new branch of technology. They are faster (up to 8.2 mph, compared with about 6 mph with others) because of very powerful motors. They do have fully adjustable controllers, however, in case the client likes the wheelchair but is unable to handle the top speeds. Their centers of gravity are lower (by about 2 to 3 inches over other wheelchairs), which allows safe maneuvering, even at top speeds. They are rigid (no parts fold or move on the main frame) and therefore potentially more durable. Recline or tilt units can be placed on these wheelchairs. Even if not used for their top speeds, the wheelchairs can be configured with a low seat height (17 inches, compared with 20 inches for other wheelchairs). This makes a big difference when a powered tilt or recline is added.

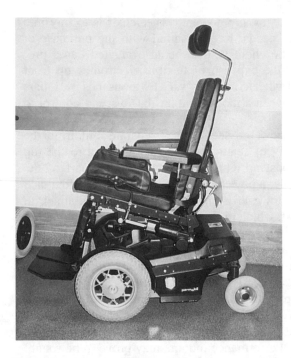

Figure 6–1. Permobil powered wheelchair.

The user will be much more accessible to his or her environment, regarding for instance, the ability to fit under tables. These wheelchairs are also shorter in the overall length, which assists with environmental accessibility.

Transportable powered wheelchairs can be taken apart and placed in a vehicle. This is not an easy process. Even when the batteries are removed, footrests and armrests are removed, and the wheelchair is folded as small as it will go, the heaviest part is still about 60 lb. The process of taking the wheelchair apart, putting it into a vehicle, and putting it back together should be demonstrated during the evaluation process so the user and any caregivers have a clear understanding of what is involved. Transportable wheelchairs have 12-inch rear wheels with 8-inch front casters. They come in two configurations: a traditional X frame, like a folding manual wheelchair, or a rigid frame styled after rigid manual wheelchairs. The rigid frames can be more durable, especially if the user is heavy (more than 200 lb) or the seat width is more than 18 inches. It has the additional advantage of having angle-adjustable backposts, which can greatly assist with positioning someone, with or without a separate back support, who cannot sit upright because of postural or balance problems.

Add-on power packs are not powered wheelchairs but systems that attach directly to the rear wheels of manual wheelchairs. A power pack is usually used when a client primarily uses a manual wheelchair but occasionally wants the benefits of powered mobility for long distances. As with a transportable powered wheelchair, the process for disassembling the unit is time consuming and not something the user is likely to be able to perform independently, because of the weight and configuration of the power pack. A power pack does well indoors and outdoors over relatively level surfaces, such as sidewalks. It is not meant or suited for rugged outdoor use. Because the motor fits directly over the rear wheel of the manual wheelchair and depends on friction to turn the wheel, conditions such as rain or a steep ramp can make it slip. When prescribing a power pack, it is a good idea to consider using it with a rigid manual wheelchair because rigid manual wheelchairs hold up better than do folding manual wheelchairs.

Scooters also come in a variety of sizes and configurations. They can be used by adults and children. They may have either front-wheel or rear-wheel drive. Usually, only the least expensive models have front-wheel drive. Front-wheel drive can be problematic, because little weight is over the front wheel of the scooter. As such, driving up a hill or ramp can leave the user without sufficient pressure on the front wheel to contact the ground, causing the scooter to lose traction. Scooters have either three or four wheels. The three-wheel scooters are most often used; they are most suited for indoor use because of the narrow front end. They are controlled with a tiller on which there are two levers on the handle bar, one for forward and one for reverse operation. The operating motion is similar to that used in turning a tricycle. The seating and positioning options on most scooters are limited. Usually, the user must be able to sit in the seat that comes with the scooter. An electric seat elevator is an option on most scooters and can help the user reach objects and change the seat height for transfers.

Scooters are appropriate for basically the same conditions as the power pack. The user of the three-wheel variety must be cautioned about turning quickly or riding on hills. These scooters can be unstable laterally if used under these conditions. Four-wheel scooters can be used under these conditions, although the user loses good indoor accessibility because of the increased front width.

Input Devices and Their Positioning

Obviously, the client has to drive the wheelchair using an input method. The method of driving chosen for the client is the most efficient and safe method for him or her. The input method has two components: the input device (e.g., joystick) and the positioning of the input device. Determining the appropriate input device is discussed later in the evaluation section.

Input methods can be divided into two categories: proportional controls and microswitch or digital controls (see pages 128–130). The types of controls that fall into these categories are discussed here. When evaluating the client, it is important to keep in mind his or her "technology tolerance," or ability to handle devices and gadgets. Some of these inputs and positioning of the inputs may require adjustment. Ensure that the client or caregiver can easily operate them.

Proportional Controls

JOYSTICK. The joystick is the most commonly used method of driving a powered wheelchair. Because it is so straightforward and technically the least complicated, the joystick should be considered first whenever the client has enough upper extremity function to use it. With the flexibility of the electronics, the travel necessary for the joystick (how far the user has to push it before the wheelchair begins to move) can be adjusted for someone with limited upper extremity range of motion. However, using a joystick can be dangerous for someone with limited upper extremity range of motion or strength (e.g., a client with a weak C-5 spinal cord injury). Overuse or trying to perform a motion that is not fully functional may feed into postural problems as the client tries to use compensatory movements. The client's posture must be carefully observed as he or she drives, particularly if spasticity involves the trunk and upper extremity, or a predominance of reflexes. Positioning of the joystick with hardware other than the standard hardware is crucial for clients with range-of-motion limitations of the shoulder (particularly rotation) and elbow. For example, if the client has a contracture in shoulder internal rotation, he or she would push the joystick in a diagonal rather than forward direction for a forward movement of the wheelchair. The therapist holds the person's forearm and asks him or her to imitate the movements necessary to move the joystick in all directions. This permits the therapist and supplier to see where the joystick needs to be mounted. They can then look at hardware to accomplish this position. Occasionally, the size of the joystick control box prohibits it from being moved where the user functions best with it. A remote joystick, which is just the joystick with the control box mounted elsewhere where the user can see it, can be used so there is more flexibility in mounting.

An individual with impaired hand or wrist musculature often uses a joystick top other than the standard ball to be able to safely and consistently move the joystick. For example, a "goalpost" configuration provides a surface on which the hand rests for forward and reverse motions and provides lips on each end for left and right motions. Depending on strength and active range of motion, the joystick and control box can be modified for the user's functional benefit. The individual's movement patterns and range of motion affect the kind of top the joystick needs.

Some individuals choose to use a joystick mounted under the chin. The advantage of this system is that the user with no upper extremity movement has direct access to a simple, proportional drive system. There are several disadvantages. First, this system places a potential strain on the cervical area. Second, many individuals do not like having the joysticks sitting in front of their faces all the time. Third, the mounting hardware has a tendency to slip slightly out of place and out of the optimal position with time.

If chin control is not desirable, there are other methods of obtaining proportional joystick control through use of the head. These methods involve using a joystick with a linkage system behind the head, so backward movement of the head runs the wheelchair forward, movement to the left runs the wheelchair to the left, and movement to the right runs the wheelchair to the right. Reverse motion is obtained by hitting a switch (any single switch) that makes the backward motion of the head reverse until the switch is hit again. These methods are appropriate for individuals who desire the feel of the proportional joystick and have good control of their heads. One problem for individuals who are using powered tilts or reclines (using them as integrated controls) is that the controls also double as the headrests. They must be able to lift their heads off the controls when tilted or reclined, so that they can change channels and resume an upright position.

HEAD CONTROL. The Peachtree Head Control (Fig. 6–2) is unique. The control looks like a rectangular headrest pad. Inside the pad are sensors that give commands to the wheelchair controller based on position of the head in relation to the pad. It is proportional in the sense that the farther away from the pad the head goes, the faster the chair goes. Not a great deal of head movement is needed, although it has to be consistent and strong enough to maintain control outdoors and over uneven surfaces. Changing modes between drive, recline, and environmental control unit (ECU) is achieved by using the head to tap a series of beeps on the pad. For example, a single tap results in the wheelchair's immediately coming to a stop. A small plate mounted where the user can see it serves as a "directory" of command beeps to remind the user of the command sequences. If the head moves too far away from the headrest, either forward or sideways, the wheelchair stops itself. This feature functions as a safety switch (or "kill" switch) in case the individual moves out of position in the wheelchair. This control works well for users who have only head control and who possess sufficient range of motion to activate the control and maneuver safely within their environments, as mentioned previously. It is usually not appropriate for people with certain cognitive impairments, such as problems with sequencing.

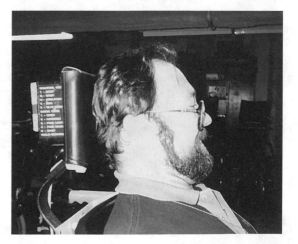

Figure   6–2. Peachtree   Head Control.

Microswitch/Digital Control

SIP AND PUFF. A Sip and Puff control works in both latched and momentary modes. The user delivers the sips and puffs through a straw that stays positioned in front of his or her mouth. The user must be able to differentiate between hard and soft sips and puffs. Each of these sips and puffs represents a command to the wheelchair controller. For example, a soft sip would be a left turn and a soft puff a right turn. Usually, forward and reverse operate in the latched mode, while left and right operate in the momentary mode. In this way, the user latches into forward motion and can make momentary course corrections to the left and right. The user can change modes to tilt or recline in two ways. One is through automatically allowing the wheelchair to go to reset, from which the user can change to the recline mode. The other is to use a separate switch as a mode switch, which also serves as a kill switch. If the user desires, the recline or tilt switch or switches can be mounted to the headrest and operated separately from the powered wheelchair system altogether, although that may make it difficult to locate a kill switch.

Sip and Puff can be somewhat difficult to introduce to a client. Not only does the client need to differentiate between soft and hard sips and puffs, but he or she must learn to sequence the commands to drive the chair. One method of teaching this is through a computer program that allows the user to practice the physical oral–motor skills and begin to use these skills on a series of "test tracks" on the computer screen. (Information on this computer software can be obtained at the Shepherd Center, Assistive Technology Center; see Appendix B.) Learning Sip and Puff techniques is an abstract skill, and any assistance the client is given to learn some of the prerequisite skills is helpful.

Single switches are another method of microswitch or digital control. Any combination of switches can be used. One switch for each direction is needed along with one switch needed as a kill switch. These switches are useful for clients who have very gross upper extremity control, such as someone with severe cerebral palsy, or with a client who has multiple sites in various places on the body (scattered control). As discussed previously, a microswitch is either on or off. This provides for a "choppy" control of the wheelchair. The clients goes forward, stops, hits the switch for a right turn, stops, hits forward again, stops. Some microswitch users learn to hit forward and right or left simultaneously to go in a diagonal direction. Generally, it is the least smooth method of driving a powered wheelchair.

Other Details of the Power System

As you may have gleaned from the previous information, any method of driving other than joystick with the hand requires a kill switch in case the control fails. In addition, if the individual is using a recline or tilt system, a separate mode-changing switch can be used. If the individual in a manual chair is using a powered tilt or recline system, a single or dual switch is used to assume a reclining position, then return to a sitting position. Usually, the switches are tape switches and are mounted on the headrest. A single switch can be used to operate both powered recline or tilt for both directions. For example, a single switch could be mounted to the headrest. An attendant control is recommended if the individual is not able to handle all driving situations, such as driving onto a van wheelchair lift. Because this is an expensive option, the function of this control must be carefully thought out to justify it to a funding agency.

Clients who require a ventilator will need a powered wheelchair that can accept a ventilator tray to handle this and any other supplies the client must carry with him or her.

Powered Mobility Evaluation

Considerations in Evaluation for Powered Mobility

It is assumed that the client has already been appropriately positioned within the wheelchair. A powered wheelchair should not be recommended if the client has not had an opportunity to drive the wheelchair. Only by observing the client drive, can the therapist determine if the client can safely operate the powered chair in various environments and if the controls are placed in the most efficient position. When evaluating, an electronically adjustable powered chair is useful so a variety of controls can be used with the same chair. A traditional powered chair or a transportable powered chair with an adjustable seat to back angle will serve clients who do not need a recline or tilt feature. A chair with powered tilt and recline may be used for those who do not need that feature so that access to recline and tilt controls and the client's positioning during recline or tilt can be assessed. Trying a variety of cushions, backs, lateral supports, and headrests will permit the therapist to appropriately position the client.

The evaluation can be broken into two main sections — activities before the evaluation, including assessing the client's best sites for physical access to the control, matching physical access to type of controls, and positioning the controls in the optimum position for access, and activities during the evaluation. Activities before the evaluation are discussed in earlier chapters. They are addressed briefly below. This chapter focuses on activities during the evaluation.

Activities Before the Evaluation

Once the client is positioned correctly, attention is directed toward identification of a control site(s) to access the input method. The client has to perform four wheelchair functions: forward, back, left, and right. The control site must offer movement that is voluntary, consistent, and repeatable. The client must be able to access and maintain access to the input control. Generally, sites are evaluated in a particular order: hands, arms, legs, head, and feet (Wright & Barker, 1993). The main reason for looking at anatomic sites in this order is that the less "technical" a powered mobility device looks, the more likely it is to be viewed as acceptable to the client, his or her caregivers, and those in the client's environments. Some of the control sites noted here require technical and expensive mounting of input switches, such as when four separate microswitches need to be mounted at four separate physical sites. The hands and arms are the most frequently used sites and the sites most often found acceptable.

Sometimes, a therapist must identify two to four sites that are functional. Some clients, especially those with cerebral palsy and severe orthopedic impairments, such as arthrogryposis, may not have one site that can move in all directions, as would be necessary with a joystick, but have separate sites on the body that can perform one movement. As with the seating evaluation, the therapist's role is to feel and observe the degree and intensity of the movements at these various sites (Wright & Barker, 1993). More information on switches and access can be found in Chapter 3.

Once the therapist has identified sites, an input method can be chosen and matched to the client's control sites. The therapist can test the efficacy of these input devices prior to driving by connecting the input method to computer games. This will allow the therapist to see if the site is truly functional once functional demands are placed on the client. It may also permit fine-tuning of the input device location. This interim step may be helpful but is not a substitute for allowing the client to drive. The actual driving portion permits clients to independently control their movements, while the therapist observes the effects of driving on the client's tone, reflexes, strength, and visual-perceptual problem-solving abilities.

Once the input method and site are determined, the client is ready to try driving. This often requires an array of hardware to allow positioning of the input control. Some facilities have adapted powered chairs with adjustable seating devices so the client can be well positioned during the seating evaluation and hardware to allow positioning of the input control (Taylor, 1986).

Activities During the Evaluation

The client should be given simple instructions on how the chair and input device work. The therapist may want to briefly demonstrate how this works (i.e., gently guiding the client's hand on the joystick). The driving should take place in as wide open a space as possible. If there are too many obstacles, the client's concerns about running into objects may hinder the therapist from receiving an accurate reflection of the client's abilities. The amount of time the client requires to try driving will vary with the client's diagnosis, age, cognitive status, and severity of physical environment.

After the initial introduction of the chair, the therapist should ensure that verbal and physical cues to the client are limited from anyone involved with the evaluation (Kangas, 1993). What could be more confusing than people constantly directing someone new to driving? The client, especially an individual with abnormal tone or reflexes and cognitive problems, needs time to determine how he or she can best use the body for the functional skill of driving. Even more important is the fact that the evaluation may be the first time the client has ever moved completely on his or her own. At first, the client may be completely disinterested in paying attention to anyone!

By the end of the evaluation, the client should demonstrate at least several basic skills:

1. Clients must be able to stop on command. This may not be entirely consistent by the end of the evaluation due to age or cognitive level.
2. Clients must be aware that their movements have an effect on movements of the wheelchair. The therapist also observes the effects the moving wheelchair has on the client. For example, some individuals with abnormal tone or reflexes may experience increased tone over rough, outdoor surfaces and lose control of the chair.
3. Clients should be able to maintain control of the input device without stopping every few feet to regain control. For example, a client with a weak C-5 spinal cord injury may be able to operate a joystick with arm support for 10 minutes but may not have sufficient strength beyond these short distances.

Of course, not every client is ready for powered mobility at the end of one evaluation session. Some require further evaluation and training sessions in more familiar environments, such as school. Depending on the client's cognitive and physical levels, environments are gradually introduced, including outdoors and busy areas. The client should be able to handle these environments with good judgment of dangers displayed (with children, within age-appropriate levels). When the client is not able to show good judgment or understanding of the powered chair, the team must decide if a powered chair is appropriate. In some cases, a powered chair may be recommended if the client will have constant care or attendant supervision.

Once the control method is determined, the client or caregiver, therapist, and supplier decide on which powered wheelchair will best meet the client's needs.

Conclusion

Choices of powered mobility technology have become overwhelming. The "match game" can be made into a more systematic process if the members of the evaluation team understand the technology and how to manipulate it. A thorough understanding of the client's physical, functional, and ADL abilities as well as the client's activity level and environments will assist the team in matching appropriate technology.

MANUAL WHEELCHAIR PERFORMANCE AND TECHNOLOGY

Finding the right manual wheelchair among the many choices means identifying a person's abilities and personal preferences and matching them with the technology that maximizes the person's potential. As with powered mobility, professionals must take the time to listen, assess, and gather information about the user. In addition, we must provide useful information about manual wheelchairs and wheelchair components to the consumer so that an educated decision can be made.

Because mobility is the primary purpose of the manual wheelchair, it is important to identify the level of the user's current wheelchair mobility skills or determine the potential for manual wheelchair propulsion. Some questions that may need to be answered (most of the necessary information will be gathered in the seating evaluation) include the following:

- Can the person propel on level surfaces only? Once a hill or uneven ground is introduced, does the person become unable to propel?
- Does the person have full upper extremity and hand function? If not, are special handrims, such as plastic-coated handrims, necessary to provide a gripping surface? Can this person stop safely on challenging terrain?
- Does the person have sufficient strength and endurance to ascend inclines?
- Will the person use his or her arms, legs, or combination of both to propel the wheelchair?
- Can the person manage steep ramps, curbs, stairs, and rough terrain? If so, what adjustments or frame designs are necessary to allow this person to perform at maximal efficiency?

The therapist must look at the ADLs that are performed while sitting in the wheelchair. For example, does the person dress, work, and perform bladder management and weight shifts? Accessibility in the home, workplace, or school may relate to wheelchair seat height, floor-to-top-of-the-knee height, and seat angle. Dressing and bladder management can influence wheelchair back height and composition. Sitting balance for all these activities may depend on orientation of the user relative to gravity and his or her posture within the wheelchair. Transfer ability and the client's general level of independence can be made better or worse depending on the design of the wheelchair and seating. Does the person require a specific seat height for transfers to and from the bed, car, or floor? Are the feet supported by the footrest during the transfer, and is a longer wheelchair base needed to prevent forward tipping? Can the feet be placed on the floor during transfers? Does the person ambulate with braces? Does his or her walking technique require footrests that swing out of the way to come to a standing position from the wheelchair (Kreutz, 1995)?

As with powered mobility, transportation issues must be examined. Does the client load the wheelchair independently, or does he or she require partial or complete assistance? Is the vehicle a two- or four-door car? What technique does the person use to load the wheelchair into the vehicle? What is the folded width and dimensions of the wheelchair and the allowable space behind the driver's seat or in the trunk of the vehicle?

Categories of Manual Wheelchairs

Manual wheelchairs can be separated into two categories: dependent transport wheelchairs and wheelchairs for independent mobility. Dependent transport wheelchairs are for people for whom independent mobility is not an option or goal. They include transport chairs, manual recliners, and manual tilt-in-space wheelchairs. Wheelchairs for independent mobility include standard heavy-duty wheelchairs, hemiheight (low seat height) wheelchairs, lightweight wheelchairs, and adjustable lightweight wheelchairs. Of course, the main purpose of independent manual wheelchairs is to provide the individual with an efficient wheelchair setup to maximize the client's physical skills.

Dependent Transport Wheelchairs

Dependent wheelchairs are available in three basic styles: standard transport, manual reclining, and manual tilt-in-space wheelchairs.

A variety of wheelchairs can function as transport wheelchairs. The true transport chair has a folding frame, four small wheels, and removable leg rests. Some also have removable armrests and a fold down back. The small four wheels allow for a small overall width compared with the style with large wheels in the rear and small wheels in the front. Standard heavy-duty wheelchairs can be used as dependent transport chairs. They offer improved durability and stability and can be pushed more easily over a variety of terrains. Loading of these wheelchairs into a car can present a problem for the caregiver, because they can be heavy, about 50 lb.

Manual Reclining Wheelchairs

Manual reclining wheelchairs are used for individuals who are unable to sit at 90 degrees at the hips and knees or in an upright position because of hypotension, contractures at the hips, or poor endurance. The recline feature also allows for dependent intermittent pressure relief. Disadvantages are weight (exceeding 60–70 lb) and overall length of the wheelchair. This can make transportation and accessibility difficult. Antitip devices should be prescribed with these chairs to prevent them from tipping over backward when reclined (Fig. 6–3).

Manual Tilt-in-Space Wheelchairs

Manual tilt-in-space wheelchairs are used for the same reasons as a manual recliner. They are used for people who have the additional complications of a fixed hip angle or fixed trunk deformities or severe spasticity when being moved from a sitting position to a supine position.

Manual Wheelchairs for Independent Mobility

Standard wheelchairs had traditionally been the most used wheelchairs of this category, but in the last 10 years, they have been replaced in large part

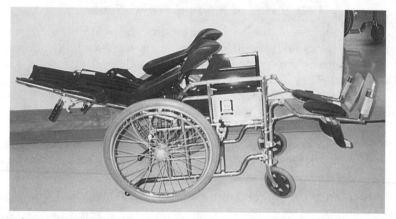

Figure 6–3. Manual reclining chair.

by more adjustable lightweight counterparts. The standard wheelchairs are used for clients who have good sitting balance and upper extremity strength but who do not want to use advanced mobility skills, such as ascending and descending curbs. Many people may not be able to load this chair because of the weight. The standard wheelchair frame is made with a crossbrace that allows it to fold. Tubing is usually low-carbon steel, although some manufacturers have used chrome or stainless steel to resist rusting. Swing away footrests, removable armrests, and sling upholstery are standard features. The disadvantages include lack of adjustability to affect wheelchair performance and weights exceeding 45 lb. Availability of dimensions and seat heights is also very limited. A standard seat height is 19 to 21 inches and hemiheight is 17 to 18 inches. A super hemiheight wheelchair is 14 to 15 inches. These lower height wheelchairs are used for the person who uses his or her lower extremities for propulsion. If the person's lower leg length is 17 inches or less and the wheelchair cushion is 2 inches or more, a seat height of anything more than 15 inches will render mobility very difficult and result in poor posture as the person slides down in the seat to be able to reach the floor. Children's sizes can vary from 8 to 16 inches wide to the same range for depth. Seat heights can vary from about 10 to 18 inches. There are no "standard" sizes for children as there traditionally are for adults.

Heavy-duty and extra-heavy-duty wheelchairs are used to support clients who weigh greater than 250 and 300 lb, respectively. Most standard, lightweight, and ultralight wheelchairs are guaranteed for users who weigh less than 250 lb. These heavy-duty and extra-heavy-duty wheelchairs can come with double cross-braces and extra frame reinforcements. Seat widths and depths can be custom made on extra-heavy-duty wheelchairs to accommodate almost any size client.

Lightweight wheelchairs have the same features as standard wheelchairs, with the exception of a weight equal to or less than 36 lb. This weight may make the difference in independent loading of a wheelchair into the vehicle but will result in little, if any, improvement in efficient wheelchair performance over the standard wheelchair.

Adjustable lightweight wheelchairs differ from the previous groups in weight (30–34 lb), some rear axle adjustability, more options for seat width and depth dimensions, and backpost height options. This wheelchair may be slightly easier to manage for independent loading into a vehicle because of decreased weight. It also allows some adjustability at the axle for tilting the seat for balance.

The final category is the adjustable ultralight wheelchair (less then 30 lb). This category is composed of folding, rigid, and custom-fitted nonadjustable wheelchairs (these are not discussed, because they are usually sport chairs). The key advantage of this group is the ability to change dimensions and characteristics of the wheelchair performance. These wheelchairs are capable of creating a higher level of user independence and performance if fitted and adjusted to the client's needs. This is the only group that allows for performance adjustments.

Personal preference should dictate the final decision about what type of adjustable, ultralight wheelchair to use. The following text covers a variety of options. Frame design is the first decision. Options are either *folding* or *rigid*. Clinical applications for a folding frame design include users who frequently encounter rough terrain and who are unable to remove the wheels and lift the wheelchair into the car. The flex in the folding frame designs helps to maintain four wheels in contact with the ground when going over rough terrain. This is essential if the user is not skilled at performing "wheelies," in which the user lifts the front wheels off the ground and balances and propels on the rear wheels. Some problems arise from this folding frame design. First, the hardware that allows for adjustability of the rear wheels also results in a folded wheelchair width of 12 to 13 inches as compared with the folding width of about 11 inches of the nonadjustable models. This may make fitting it behind the driver's seat nearly impossible. Some of the newest chairs are reducing the widths to approximately 11 inches. The other problem is that these folding frames have more flex in the frame, which results in poorer efficiency and more energy being put into propulsion on the user's part. One advantage of the folding frame is the ability to change seat width by changing the cross-frame in case the user gains or loses weight.

Rigid frames, when compared with folding frames, offer advantages of better translation of energy and responsiveness of the wheelchair to the user, greater durability because of less flex in the frame, and smaller turning radius and back angle adjustment. Methods of adjusting the performance of the wheelchair vary significantly between brands. Some adjustments may require purchase of additional components. It is important to determine the optimal position and adjustment prior to ordering the wheelchair so only components that are necessary are purchased.

Components of Wheelchairs

Frame Materials

Wheelchairs are made of a variety of materials. Not all features and components are available for all types of wheelchairs. As previously mentioned, the adjustable, ultralight wheelchair offers the most choices for features and function. Aluminum is the most common, but chromoly, steel, titanium, and carbon fiber composite are also options. Strength is an important issue, but nearly all these frames have lifetime guarantees unless abused. Another consideration is the shock absorption characteristics of the different metals. The new carbon fiber frames (same technology used with racing bicycles) dampen vibration and absorb shock the best.

Rear Wheels

Rear wheels are either spoke or molded plastic (Fig. 6–4). In the wheels of the chair, the greatest effects on propulsion can be realized. The less the wheel weighs, the less work the user must do to overcome inertia. Another way of improving propulsion efficiency is by increasing the wheel stiffness. The advantage of a mag wheel is that it is essentially maintenance free. However, mag wheels are heavier than spoke wheels. They also have a greater degree of lateral flex, which results in less efficiency during propulsion.

Rear Tires

Tires for wheelchairs are either pneumatic (air-filled) or solid. Pneumatic tires vary in their material composition, profile (i.e., treaded, nontreaded), size,

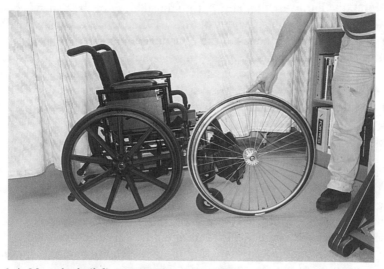

Figure 6–4. Mag wheels (*left*) versus spoke wheels (*right*).

and recommended maximum pressure. When comparing rollability of tires on a hard surface, the sequence of tires from best to worst would be as follows: high pressure tires (120 lb per square inch [PSI]), standard pneumatics (55–60 PSI), solid tires, and pneumatic tires with solid inserts. As tire pressure decreases, rolling resistance increases. Pneumatic tires also absorb shock better than solid tires, giving a smoother ride. The flip side of the coin is durability. Solid tires far outlast pneumatic tires.

Standard tire size is 24 inches in diameter. However, 20-, 22- and 26-inch wheels are also used. Tire size usually correlates to client arm length. For example, many children and adults with spina bifida have very long arms and a shortened trunk. The 22-inch wheels with a smaller diameter could be more efficient.

Axle

Rear wheel axles are all quick release on adjustable ultralight wheelchairs. Some offer an extension on the quick release mechanism that allows someone with minimal hand function to release the lock and remove the wheel. All are able to be moved anteriorly and posteriorly to affect center of gravity (tippiness) of the chair up and down to affect tilt of the chair.

Casters

Just like rear tires, casters come in a variety of sizes, profiles, and materials. Some important facts must be considered when deciding on the type of caster. First, the appropriate size caster for propulsion is determined. Casters vary in size from 8 inches in diameter to 3-inch rollers (same size and type as used with in-line skates). Sizes vary depending on the client's functional skills and environment. Larger caster wheels make it easier to push the wheelchair over obstacles. This is especially important if the person is unable to perform a wheelie. The caster must also be selected to reduce caster flutter, which is an abrupt stop or change in direction for rider safety. Caster flutter occurs when the casters are not making good contact with the ground and start shaking. The feeling is similar to when your front wheels are out of alignment on your car. Thacker, Sprigle, and Morris (1994), identified four factors that reduce caster flutter:

- Using lighter or smaller caster wheels
- Increasing the trail length (perpendicular distance from caster stem to point of contact of the caster)
- Increasing the stem axle friction
- Having the caster stem perpendicular to the ground

In addition to the factors regarding safe mobility, comfort and positioning concerns must be considered when deciding on the appropriate casters. Pneumatic casters provide a much smoother ride than solid casters. Unfortunately, maintenance is a real problem, because they constantly require being filled with air. How often will vary depending on the client's activity level. Some hybrid casters combine the feel of pneumatic with the durability of solid tires. Caster pin locks may be necessary to lock the casters in a forward-facing position for transferring for individuals who have borderline transfer skills, because they keep the casters from turning while the person transfers to or from the wheelchair. Finally, caster size and footrest angles must be considered simultaneously. Knee flexion contractures can result in the knee needing to be positioned close to 90 degrees. This would require reducing the caster trail and size to accommodate these contractures. Reducing caster trail lessens the amount of space the caster travels as it turns so that it is less likely to contact the individual's foot as it turns.

Armrest

Armrests vary in design and use. Sometimes they serve as upper extremity support for clients with little or no upper extremity function. Most wheelchairs have the option of armrests that provide adjustment in height (Fig. 6–5). Arm supports, such as arm troughs and trays, can be mounted to these armrests.

Operation of different armrest styles can vary from requiring only wrist control to requiring excellent dexterity in both upper extremities. Flip-back design operation or tubular swing away are easily manageable by a person with limited hand function.

Footrest

Footrests may be fixed angle, swing away, or rigid nonremovable, straight, or tapered. Elevating leg rests are applicable if the person has a knee extension contracture or severe hypotension.

Fixed-angle footrests, which can be swing away or rigid, vary from 60 degrees to 90 degrees. The larger the angle of the footrest the greater the

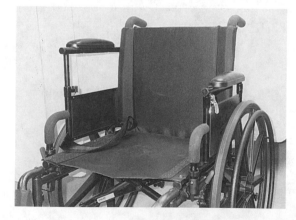

Figure 6–5. Example of adjustable-height arms.

degree of knee flexion that can be obtained. The greater the knee flexion, the shorter the overall wheelchair frame length. As knee flexion is increased, ground and caster clearance must not become problems.

Foot plates can also provide accommodations for varying angles of ankle flexion.

Manual Wheelchair Performance

The factors that affect performance of a wheelchair will be grouped according to their impact on the maneuverability of the wheelchair. This section attempts to explain the factors and their implications on wheelchair propulsion, safety, and energy expenditure.

Rolling Resistance

The setup of a wheelchair dictates how it will respond to the actions of the user. This section begins with the issue of rolling resistance. A client who pushes a manual wheelchair must overcome the resistance to movement of the wheelchair caused by friction. With wheelchair propulsion, friction can be affected by tire size and composition, tire pressure, wheel alignment, wheel bearings, ground surface, and aerodynamics (O'Reagan et al., 1981). The greater the contact between the tire and the ground, the greater the friction or rolling resistance. If a user were rolling on mountain bike tires, the resistance would be greater than if he or she were using racing bike tires. This resistance may mean the difference between independent and dependent or very inefficient propulsion for the user with impaired strength and function in the upper extremities. Even for the user with normal upper extremity strength, increased friction will mean a greater expenditure of energy to make the chair roll.

As stated previously, friction is affected by many different factors. Tire design should be selected based on the type of terrain the client will be primarily encountering. The harder the ground surface, the smaller the tire radius, or "footprint," needs to be to reduce friction. Small-profile tires are more effective in reducing rolling resistance on hard surfaces. Conversely, large-profile tires reduce friction on softer ground and sandy soils (Hofstad & Patterson, 1994).

Wheel and frame alignment also affect rolling resistance. Wheel and frame alignment that results in "toe in" or "toe out" causes significant drag on the wheel as the wheelchair is pushed, almost like that created by a skier bringing the tips of the skis together to snow plow down the ski slope to increase friction and slow down. Wheel alignment is easily tested by measuring the distance between the two rims at the height of the axle from the floor in the front and the rear of the chair. The distance between the rims at the front and the back should be equal (Shepherd, 1992). This means that the wheels are parallel and will not "plow" the surface they are negotiating. Frame alignment and wheel alignment can impact toe in and toe out. Rigid frame wheelchairs are less likely to create this condition than folding frame manual wheelchairs because of the increased flex in the frame. Testing for toe in and toe out should be done if the axle position is altered.

Friction can be useful with some wheelchairs under some conditions. One condition is when a user with impaired hand and upper extremity function uses plastic-coated handrims, foam handrims, or knobs on the handrims. This increases friction at the handrims to make up for loss of upper extremity or hand function. Safety may be one reason to increase rolling resistance under some environmental situations. For example, larger profile (wider) tires or tires with more substantial tread can prevent a user from losing control when descending a wet or steep ramp.

Maneuverability

Maneuverability is another aspect of wheelchair performance. Maneuverability is how the wheelchair responds to the user's actions. Wheel composition, frame composition and design, the combined weight of the wheelchair and user, and the distribution of the weight of the user in the wheelchair all influence how the wheelchair responds to the user's push.

The factor that has the greatest impact on maneuverability and control of the wheelchair is the distribution of weight of the user relative to the rear wheel axle (Fig. 6–6). The closer the center of gravity of the user is to the

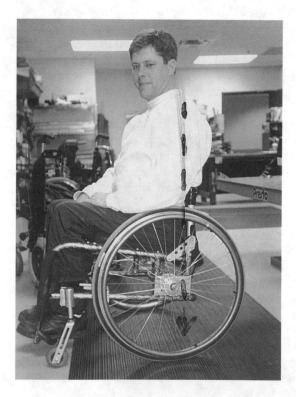

Figure 6–6. Notice that the bulk of the user's weight falls behind the axle, increasing responsiveness and tippiness.

rear wheel axle, the easier the wheelchair is to turn (Shepherd, 1992). This unloads the front casters and results in a decrease in the wheelchair's tendency to turn downhill when a wheelchair user traverses a slope. Pushing a wheelchair on a sidewalk is a good example, because nearly all sidewalks are constructed to slope toward the street. The user, in this situation, must apply more effort with the upper extremity on the street side to track a straighter line and keep from rolling into the street.

Moving the center of gravity of the user rearward and upward over the rear axle results in better control in the wheelie position (Fig. 6–7). This improves *dynamic* mobility, making such skills as ascending curbs, descending ramps, and propelling over rough terrain easier. The disadvantage to this rearward distribution of the user's center of gravity is a loss of *static* stability. For example, the wheelchair is easier to tip over backward if the user leans backward (especially abruptly) or attempts to start pushing up an incline without leaning forward. Good upper extremity strength and trunk balance are necessary.

Lateral Stability

Another performance issue is the lateral stability of the wheelchair. In contrast with the higher seat position for ease of wheelies, a lower seat height is recommended to prevent tipping of the wheelchair sideways. Adding to the wheels is one method of increasing the wheelchair's lateral stability. Camber makes the base of support wider by angling out the wheels at the bottom, which then angles them in at the top. There are some functional reasons for adding camber to the wheelchair: better access to the tire and handrim for propulsion and a propulsion stroke of the upper extremities moving in a downward and outward direction that is more natural. Different manufacturers use significantly different methods to change camber (Fig. 6–8).

One sacrifice as a result of adding camber is an increase in the overall and folded and unfolded widths of the wheelchair, which can significantly

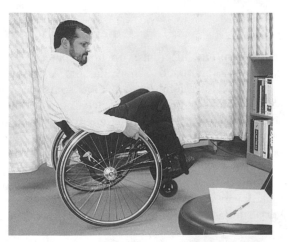

Figure 6–7. Moving the wheels forward results in a better wheelie position.

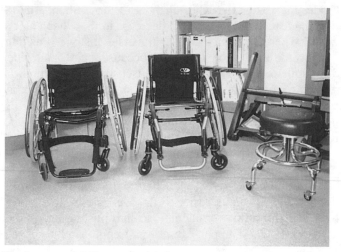

Figure 6–8. Camber on a rigid-frame wheelchair.

limit accessibility. For example, adding 6 degrees of camber to a 16-inch-wide seat increases the overall width of the chair from approximately 24 to 29 inches. Standard doorways are usually 30 inches.

Just as with powered mobility, selecting a manual wheelchair's performance characteristics is a compromise of numerous decisions. Improving maneuverability is important because the majority of wheelchair activities are of short duration and involve continuous changes in direction. Prescribing a lightweight wheelchair makes the wheelchair easier for the individual to load. This *adjustability* of performance is the justification for lightweight wheelchairs. Prescribing a standard heavy-duty nonadjustable wheelchair for an active client can inhibit him or her by requiring greater energy expenditure or limiting the ability to perform certain activities altogether. Functional outcomes should be the determining factor in the justification of a specific wheelchair for every user.

Other Considerations

There are differences in how someone with a long-standing injury or condition is approached in evaluation. A person who has been using a certain wheelchair for a long time, such as someone who had polio, has gotten used to functioning within that wheelchair environment. Usually, the wheelchair is set up to work with all of the environments in which the individual interacts on a regular basis. Trying to change this can often result in drastically altering or eliminating independence in certain ADL or functional skills.

If the client decides to change, his or her goals and a thorough understanding of how he or she functions is absolutely necessary. It is also a good idea, whenever possible, to have the RTS take the recommended chair, or one very similar, to the client's home, work, or school.

When measuring someone for a manual or powered chair, it is best to have them simulated in the same or similar chair to what is being recommended in the desired seated posture. The basic measurements are the same as that for a seating evaluation, with particular attention paid to lower leg length for foot and footrest clearance.

Children and people with progressive conditions are steered toward wheelchairs that offer ready growth and change. The therapist should be aware of how these changes are accomplished, about how much the changes cost, and how they are accomplished to inform the client and caregiver for their future reference.

Adapted Strollers

Sometimes infants and children use adapted stroller bases rather than manual wheelchairs. This usually offers an adapted car seat for safety, which can be attached to a stroller for parent convenience. Some stroller bases are strong enough to handle attachments for ventilators for ventilator-dependent children. Many are also crash-tested and can be tied down in vans and buses. The therapist must be careful when recommending a stroller. A child who has the ability to use a manual or powered wheelchair will be completely dependent in a stroller. Also, the therapist must ensure that the child has a few years of growing room. Most funding agencies want a wheelchair or stroller to last between 3 and 5 years before they will purchase a new one.

FUNDING ISSUES

Funding issues are basically the same for wheelchairs as they are for seating. It is best to work with the RTS, who should be well versed in the information necessary for each funding agency. Each funding agency, insurance company, Medicaid (state funding), and Medicare (federal funding for elderly and disabled individuals) has specific rules and equipment they will and will not provide. The therapist must list the desired equipment and functionally justify why it is necessary. Funding is discussed in greater detail in Chapter 10. Two sample letters of medical necessity are included as a reference (Appendix A).

Case Study

Trisha

Trisha is a 19-year-old woman with cerebral palsy since birth. She was seen by the seating and mobility clinic to determine the most appropriate equipment for her. She has a custom-molded seating system, which she has had for 5 years. This no longer fits. Overall, the width of her present wheelchair is 26 ½ inches. Her home environment is accessible to this width. It is a standard, upright wheelchair. In addition to the seating system not fitting, her mother has expressed a desire to provide Trisha with a wheelchair that changes position in space so she can have a choice of positions throughout the day.

Trisha does not have a significant medical history. She has had several orthopedic surgeries. These include the repair of a left dislocated hip with adductor releases, bilateral hamstring releases, and a spinal fusion. The hip repair left her with a shortened left femoral area.

Trisha has a scoliotic posture (spine was fused in about 30 degrees of scoliosis), with a pelvic obliquity to the left (Fig. 6–9). She also has a fixed lordotic posture (Fig. 6–10), her hips are in a "windblown" posture to the right (Figs. 6–11 and 6–12). Her hamstrings are very tight, necessitating knees being positioned at greater than 90 degrees.

Trisha has normal sensation, but is very bony in the coccygeal area. This area is prone to skin breakdown.

Trisha is generally hypotonic throughout. She has mild flexor tone in her lower extremities, with increased flexion and external rotation at the shoulder and flexion at the elbow. She tends to go into this upper extremity posture when she feels poorly supported or insecure.

Environmentally, Trisha's home is completely accessible. The family has a full-size van with tie-downs for the wheelchair. TL attends public school and is transported to school on a bus with a lift. The school is also accessible.

Trisha has good head control but no trunk balance. She is nonverbal but does respond to yes or no questions and makes it known when she is not happy with something. She does have an electronic augmentative

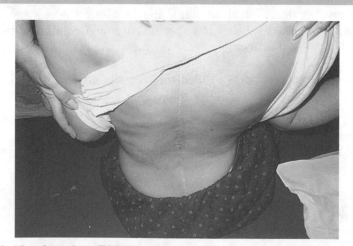

Figure 6–9. View from above Trisha's assymmetrical trunk.

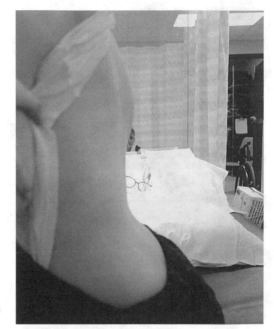

Figure 6–10. Lateral view of Trisha's lordosis.

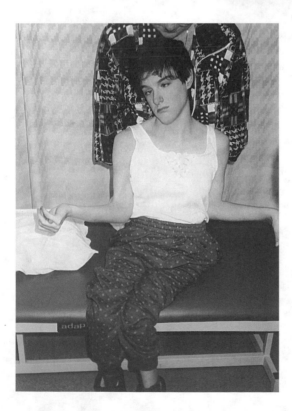

Figure 6–11. Trisha with posterior pelvis and some trunk support on the mat. Note the windblown position of the lower extremities.

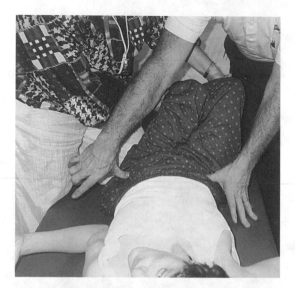

Figure 6–12. Palpating anterior superior iliac spines in supine. Note the ASIS's are facing forward, while allowing the lower extremities to remain windblown.

communication device but does not use it regularly. There is a mounting device for it, which will have to be transferred to a new wheelchair. She accesses this device with a head pointer.

Trisha was evaluated in a seating simulator that provided custom-contoured simulation. From the mold made from the simulator, seating components will be made by the manufacturer (Pin Dot Products); (Fig. 6–13). Trisha's family has private insurance, which will cover this seating system and wheelchair at 100%.

Final goals are provided in Table 6–1.

Table 6–1. FINAL GOALS FOR TRISHA

Area	Goal	Solution
Pelvis	Accommodate windblown hips to allow forward-facing trunk and head; provide anterior pelvic support to stabilize pelvis	Contour-U seat Padded lap belt
Lower extremities	Accommodate windblown hips and tight hamstrings; allow greater than 90 degrees at the hips	Same as above plus angle-adjustable leg rests
Trunk	Accommodate trunk asymmetries. Provide aggressive lateral thoracic support for maximal stability. Accommodate bony coccyx	Contour-U back, with special attention paid to coccygeal area—relieve and use closed-cell Roho mini cells (air-filled cells) in the relieved area

Table 6–1. FINAL GOALS FOR TRISHA (*Continued*)

Area	Goal	Solution
Head	Provide posterior head support for transportation	Already has a headrest, which will be reused
Mobility	Provide wheelchair that tilts in space to allow change of position throughout the day. This will be done by a caregiver	Quickie tilt-in-space manual wheelchair

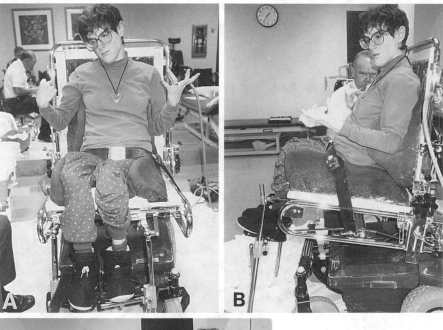

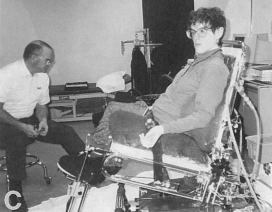

Figure 6–13. *A–C,* Trisha in adapted wheelchair. Note how Trisha's upper extremities relax as she feels more comfortable and stable. Also note in *A* the forward-facing head and trunk.

Case Study

Paul

Paul is a 27-year-old man with a 5-year history of multiple sclerosis (MS). He recently had an exacerbation, which left him unable to ambulate. Paul is blind secondary to the MS. The blindness has been present for about 1½ years.

Paul's present equipment consists of a standard manual wheelchair, which was on loan to him until his own chair could be obtained (Fig. 6–14). He states that he is able to use this wheelchair within his home independently because the environment is familiar.

Paul has had no relevant surgeries. Orthopedic status consists of a postural posteriorly tilted pelvis with a concomitant kyphotic posture (Fig. 6–15). This is primarily from trunk muscular weakness. His hamstrings are tight, necessitating a 90-degree angle at the knees to decrease the pull of the hamstrings on the pelvis into posterior pelvic tilt. Neuromotor status consists of mild flexor tone in the lower extremities, which feeds into the tight hamstrings. Additionally, his trunk is mildly low tone.

Paul has impaired sensation over his buttocks and lower extremities. This puts him at risk for the development of pressure sores.

Paul uses a transport service (van with a lift and tie-downs). He receives help from his family for ADLs, although he states that he is independent in his home because it is a familiar environment. He is not currently employed. Paul has Medicaid, which covered the cost of the chair and seating.

Final goals for Paul are provided in Table 6–2.

Table 6–2. FINAL GOALS FOR PAUL

Area	Goal	Solution
Pelvis	Provide midline, stable pelvis; decrease tendency to fall into posterior tilt by providing posterior pelvic support Accommodate impaired sensation by providing pressure-relieving cushion	Jay cushion with wood insert inside the cushion cover to maintain stability

Table 6–2. FINAL GOALS FOR PAUL (*Continued*)

Area	Goal	Solution
Lower extremities	Accommodate tight hamstrings by allowing knees to position as close to 90 degrees as possible	70-degree footrests, which because of his height, allow a 90-degree angle
Trunk	Provide posterior trunk support to decrease kyphotic posture and accommodate for weakness in trunk	Jay Active back support, which contacts the posterior pelvis, putting it in a neutral position and decreasing the kyphotic posture
Mobility	Provide manual mobility, that is adjustable and lightweight (in category of an ultralightweight wheelchair) (Figs. 6–16 and 6–17). Adjustment needed because MS can result in physical changes	Quickie 2 wheelchair with 2 inches of built-in tilt to allow gravity to assist with obtaining an upright (less kyphotic) trunk posture

STUDY QUESTIONS

1. What factors would support the use of powered mobility for a pre-school-aged child? Would these differ from those for a school-aged child? What would you need to consider when looking into powered mobility for a young adult preparing to attend college? For an elderly individual entering a nursing home?

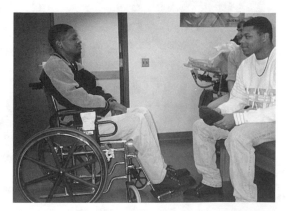

Figure 6–14. Paul in a loaner chair. Note slumped posture. Also note how far rearward the rear wheel is.

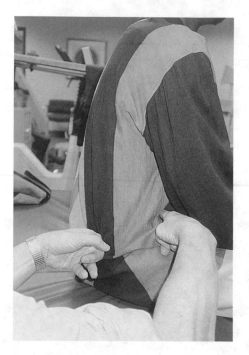

Figure 6–15. Paul sitting on a mat. Note overall rounded posture when unsupported and posterior pelvic tilt. Note that posterior superior iliac spines are down and anterior superior iliac spines are up.

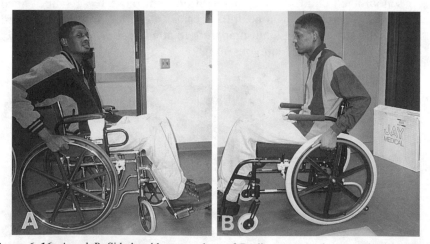

Figure 6–16. *A* and *B*. Side-by-side comparison of Paul's access to the rear wheels. With the adjustability in the new wheelchair, the wheels can be placed in an efficient position. In *B*, note the upright trunk position.

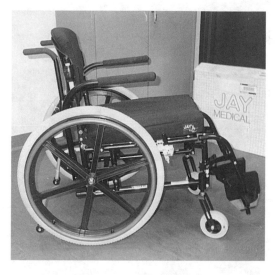

Figure 6–17. Lateral view of the chair. Note the slight tilt of the chair to assist with trunk posture.

2. What factors would you need to take into account when deciding between a standard manual wheelchair, and a lightweight manual wheelchair for an adult?

ACKNOWLEDGMENT

Special thanks to Dennis Hysong, rehabilitation equipment specialist at the Shepherd Center, for his assistance on the technical aspects of powered wheelchairs.

REFERENCES

Butler, C. (1988). High tech tots: Technology for mobility, manipulation, communication and learning in early childhood. *Infants and Young Children, 1988, 1*(2), 66–67.

Butler, C. (1991). Augmentative mobility: Why do it? *Physical Medicine and Rehabilitation Clinics of North America, 2*(4), 801–815.

Butler, C., Okamoto, G. A. & McKay, T (1983). Powered mobility for very young children. *Developmental Medicine and Child Neurology, 25,* 472–472.

Caves, K. (1994). *Introduction to integrated control systems.* Vancouver, British Columbia: Proceedings of the Tenth International Seating Symposium.

Hofstad, M. & Patterson, P. (1994). Modelling the propulsion characteristics of a standard wheelchair. *Journal of Rehabilitation Research Development, 31*(2), 129–137.

Kangas, K. (1993). *Assessment and treatment strategies for pediatric powered mobility.* Memphis, TN: Proceedings of the Ninth International Seating Symposium.

Kreutz, D. (1995). Manual wheelchairs. *Topics in Spinal Cord Injury Rehabilitation 1*(1), 1–16.

O'Reagan, J.R., Thacker, J.G., Kauzlarich, J.J., Mochel E., Carmine, D., & Bryant, M. (1981). Rolling resistance. In *Wheelchair mobility 1976-1981* (pp. 31–41). Charlottesville, VA: University of Virginia Rehabilitation Engineering Center.

Paulsson, K. & Christofferson, M. (1984). *Psycho-social aspects of technical aids: How does independent mobility affect psychological and intellectual development of children with physical disabilities?* Ottawa, Ontario: Proceedings of the Second International Conference on Rehabilitative Engineering.

Pentland, W. (1992). The weight bearing arm. *New Mobility, Summer 1992,* 41.

Shepherd, M. (1992). Performance: Tuning your lightweight wheelchair. *Action Digest, July/August*, 6–7.

Taylor, S.J. (1986). A powered mobility evaluation system. In E. Trefler, E.K. Kozole, K. & E. Snell (Ed.); *Selected readings on powered mobility for children and adults with severe physical disabilities* (pp. 69–70). Washington, DC: Resna

Taylor, S.J. (1995). Powered mobility evaluation and technology. *Topics in Spinal Cord Injury Rehabilitation* 1(1), 22–36.

Taylor, S.J. & Kreutz, D. (1994). Manual or powered mobility: What works, what doesn't. *Advance for Directors in Rehabilitation, 3*(10), 23.

Thacker, J. Sprigle, S. & Morris, B. (1994). Understanding technology when prescribing wheelchairs. Washington, DC: Resna.

Wright, C., & Barker, P. (193). *Notes from the instructional course, "Mobility experiences for young children."* Las Vegas, NV: Resna Conference.

Sample Letters of Medical Necessity

Sample 1: BJ
June 6, 1995

To Whom It May Concern:

BJ is a 32-year-old man who suffered a closed head injury as a result of a motor vehicle accident in September of 1988. BJ underwent a right frontal lobectomy with evacuation of an intracranial hematoma. Following surgery, he suffered recurrent seizures. Following his initial injury and acute hospital stay, BJ has been involved in several rehabilitation programs. He is currently unable to communicate verbally but does communicate with the assistance of a letter board. BJ is also on gastric tube feedings because of difficulty with swallowing and a history of pneumonia.

Physically, he presents with severe weakness and uncontrolled movement in all four extremities. BJ is not able to ambulate and has used a powered wheelchair for mobility since sometime in 1990. BJ is modified independent when driving this wheelchair. Because of severe intention tremors and pathological movement patterns, BJ requires a wheelchair that has the forward and turn speeds, sensitivity to joystick movement, and acceleration and torque adjusted in order to drive it safely. In tight spaces, he does have some difficulty steering the chair because of an increase in muscle tone and loss of fine motor control.

This increase in uncontrolled muscle activity is most noticeable in his right upper extremity. BJ is unable to stabilize his arm, and tremor-like movements become more prominent during volitional activities. The influence of these types of movements on controlling the wheelchair can be controlled provided the sensitivity of the joystick can be reduced. BJ's lower extremities go into extension and his left upper extremity becomes rigid in a typical hemiplegic flexed posture. The lower extremities must be restrained with positioning straps to maintain a flexed and more stable posture through the trunk and lower extremities while operating the powered wheelchair.

BJ's transfers are also influenced by the wheelchair. He requires moderate assistance. His ability to transfer is somewhat affected by the height of the surfaces he is transferring to and from. The current wheelchair has a seat height of approximately 23 inches and prevents BJ from reaching the ground with his feet to perform transfers. In coming to stand, BJ is dependent on others to release the ankle and pelvic positioning straps, assist him in coming to the front edge of the seat, and assist with the pivot itself. Standing is primarily achieved through use of significant extensor tone in his lower extremities.

In getting into the wheelchair, BJ must first sit on the edge of the wheelchair then have his feet placed on the footrests in order to push back into the seat. This places a great deal of strain on the footrests and has caused them to break numerous times.

BJ's current wheelchair is 5 years old. There are numerous mechanical problems with this wheelchair (tires, footrest failure, limited module control for smoother operation, and motor pulley wear). These problems, in addition to the interference with functional activities BJ performs, necessitate a replacement of the current equipment. Setup and trial of the following equipment took place in the Seating and Mobility Clinic at Shepherd Center on two separate occasions. BJ was independent in mobility using this equipment and could perform stand pivot transfers with less assistance.

Please find a detailed list of equipment for your client listed below:

Invacare Storm Arrow Powered Wheelchair:

Your client, BJ, must have a powered wheelchair because the amount of paralysis in his arms limits what he is able to do. While he has some residual function in his arms, his hands are paralyzed. Thus, he has no dexterity to maneuver a manual wheelchair or the strength to push a manual wheelchair for distances or on outside surfaces. The goal of your client's rehabilitation program is to return the client back to the highest level of independence. The powered wheelchair allows your client independent access to his environment.

This wheelchair must have an accompanying battery and battery charger in order to function. Heavy-duty upholstery and wheels are needed to support the weight of the patient and the chair and also to ensure durability of the chair.

Other items specified on the wheelchair are necessary to position body parts and for safety in transferring your client to and from the wheelchair. These items are described below.

- Detachable armrests and leg rests allow the patient to be moved in and out of the wheelchair more safely by allowing the chair to sit closely to other surfaces.

- Removable height-adjustable desk arms allow your client to use this chair at a desk or table. They also make transfers safer.

- Wheel locks hold the chair securely for transfers.

- The antitip levers prevent the chair from tipping over and thereby prevent injuries to your client.

Padded heavy-duty positioning belts. A pelvic positioning belt must be placed at a 70-degree angle from the seat to inhibit severe extensor tone in the trunk and provide stability at the pelvis and spine for distal extremity function. Padded 45-degree ankle straps must also be installed on each footrest to inhibit extensor tone in the legs.

Heavy-duty reinforced-angle adjustable footplates with spring-loaded extension tubes. These footrests are perhaps the most critical feature of the entire wheelchair. If they are not correct, maintaining BJ's position for operation of the wheelchair will be almost impossible. The footrest must be angle adjustable to accommodate ankle contractures. The heavy-duty version is necessary because of the severe extensor tone and history of multiple failures on the original wheelchair. The spring-loaded leg rest fittings absorb the forces from BJ's uncontrolled movement and prevent failure of the entire leg rest.

Jobst Hydrofloat Cushion:

Patient is very diaphoretic. He currently sits in a pool of perspiration all the time. This chronic perspiration can result in skin sores. The Jobst Hydrofloat cushion was used for 2 weeks by BJ and proved effective in lowering the temperature of the seating surface and thereby reducing the perspiration.

Custom Molded Back:

Your client has a diagnosis of closed head injury. This condition results in paralysis of the spinal musculature, poor sitting balance, and poor trunk stability. These problems lead to kyphotic and scoliotic sitting postures. The custom back is necessary to prevent spinal deformity and respiratory complications. In addition, this custom molded back is medically necessary to relieve pressure over your client's bony prominences to prevent skin compromise. Failure to provide this back support will result in skin breakdown.

Your immediate attention to these items that are essential to your client's continued health and independence is appreciated.

Sincerely,

DL, M.D.

JK, P.T.
Enclosure

Sample 2: AP

July 11, 1995

To Whom It May Concern:

Your client, AP, is a 9-year-old girl with spastic quadriplegic cerebral palsy. She was evaluated in the Seating and Mobility Clinic on July 6, 1995.

AP displays moderate to severe extensor tone, which also causes rotation at the pelvis. She has a pelvic obliquity to the left, with rotation to the left. She has a windblown posture of her lower extremities, with the right hip in abduction and the left in adduction. The left is shorter than the right by about 3 inches. Hamstrings are tight bilaterally. She has bilateral plantarflexion tightness. She has a scoliosis, convex to the right with a rotational component. She has fair head control, but no trunk control.

AP was evaluated in trial equipment (a seating simulator) once her physical evaluation was completed. (Please refer to the two enclosed pictures.) Results of that evaluation are as follows.

AREA	PROBLEM	GOAL	SOLUTION
Pelvis	Rotated to left; oblique to left; very bony	Accommodate all postures to provide total body support and avoid the development of decubitus ulcers	Contour-U seat (growth cushion); undercut front edge for lower extremities; body point 1-inch padded lap belt
Lower Extremities	Left dislocated hip; abduction right (windswept to right); tight hamstrings bilaterally		Pin Dot multiadjustable footrests with straps
Trunk	S-curve in spine; lordotic; no control		Contour-U back; reinforced laterals; arm relief; body point chest harness
Upper Extremities	Upper extensor tone		Clear anterior upper extremity support
Head	Fair control		Otto Bock combination headrest
Orientation in Space	Unable to sit upright; needs to be able to change positions throughout the day		Quickie Zippie tilt-n-space manual wheelchair with height-adjustable arms
Mobility	Dependent		

Should you have any concerns regarding these recommendations, please call the Seating Clinic at 350-7759.

AP's current environment and transportation are accessible. Her height is 52 inches and weight 55 pounds.

Sincerely,

DA, M.D.

MJ, OTR
Enclosure

Resources

The book *Childhood Powered Mobility: Developmental, Technical and Clinical Perspectives* is undergoing revisions and should be available sometime in 1996 through Resna Press. Resna's phone number is (703) 524-6686. Address is 1700 North Moore Street, Suite 1540, Arlington, VA, 22209-1903.

Resna is developing a certification program and examination for assistive technology providers (clinicians) and rehablitation technology suppliers. For information, please contact Resna.

Resna also sells the American National Standards Institute/Resna Wheelchair Standards book. This book provides wheelchair testing information in a standardized manner so clinicians can compare durability of chairs between brands.

The National Registry of Rehabilitation Technology Suppliers can provide you with a list of suppliers in your area who are members. They are developing a certification examination. Their address is 3223 South Loop 289, Suite 600, Lubbock, TX 79423; (806) 797-7299.

Information on the sip and puff software can be obtained from the Shepherd Center, Assistive Technology Center 2020 Peachtree Rd., Atlanta, GA 30309; Attn: John Anschutz; (404) 350-7720.

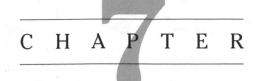

CHAPTER 7

WRITTEN AND SPOKEN AUGMENTATIVE COMMUNICATION

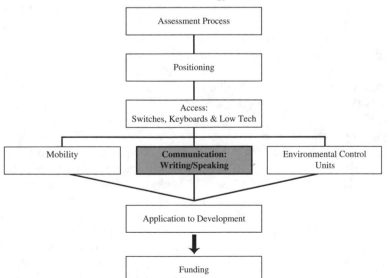

Communication is critical to everyone at every stage of life. From the moment we are born, we start to communicate with others to make our needs known. All sorts of methods to communicate are used. First, we use our voice and gross gestures. Later, these early methods are refined into language skills, facial expressions, and gestures. Some people with disabilities have difficulty developing the more refined skills. As they grow, they continue to have thoughts they want to communicate; however, it is difficult for them to convey their ideas to others. Some people with disabilities have difficulty communicating only when the communication partner is an unfamiliar listener who does not understand their particular communication style. Others are unable to communicate even with people who know them and their communication style well. When communication breakdown occurs, regardless if the partner is familiar with the communication style or not, additional time must be spent to repair the breakdown and continue the conversation. This can be frustrating to the person doing the communicating and to the communication partner. This can affect the person's ability to interact at work, school, and recreation.

Augmentative and alternative communication (AAC) is a term often associated with assistive technology (AT) and communication. The American Speech-Language-Hearing Association (ASHA) uses the following definition for AAC:

> Augmentative and alternative communication is an area of clinical practice that attempts to compensate (either temporarily or permanently) for the impairment and disability patterns of individuals with severe expressive disorders (i.e., the severely speech-language and writing impaired) (ASHA, 1989).

This chapter does not address the multimodel aspects of augmentative communication but provides information pertinent to the occupational or physical therapist working as a team member in this area. For purposes of organization, communication systems have been divided into written and spoken. Many occupational therapists and physical therapists have a broader knowledge base in written than in spoken communication. They are familiar with alternative keyboards (keyboards that are smaller or larger than the standard ones), virtual keyboards (keyboards on the computer screen), or software that can improve text entry.

Typically a team is used to assess the needs of potential AAC users. The AT guide (on p. 159) shows at what point therapists assess communication abilities. When engaged in augmentative communication assessments, a speech and language pathologist with a background in AAC is usually the team leader. Other team players can include, but are not limited to, professionals described in Chapter 1. If the client is a child, usually the team consists of a speech and language pathologist, educator, occupational therapist, seating and positioning specialist, and the parent. If the client is an adult, a typical team would be the speech and language pathologist, occupational therapist, an advocate for the client, a seating and positioning specialist, and perhaps a funding specialist. The speech and language pathologist will evaluate language capabilities, appropriate symbol sets when necessary, and particular augmentative communication devices that may be appropriate for the client's cognitive and developmental level. Occupational therapists may be responsible for evaluating the client's seating and positioning needs, motor access, visual perception, and positioning of the device for best access; integrating the augmentative communication device with the wheelchair; and determining the need for low-technology devices, such as mouth sticks, head-mounted pointers, or handheld typing tools. At times the occupational therapist finds funding for the purchase of devices that are recommended. In other clinics, it may be the physical therapist's job to evaluate seating and positioning.

Augmentative communication is typically used in a variety of settings. The school setting where children with disabilities need assistance in their communication skills may be the most prominent place augmentative communication is used. Augmentative communication is also found in rehabilitation settings where people are learning new ways to communicate following an injury or disease process. The use of augmentative communication in hospital intensive care units has been mentioned previously. Additionally, people are using augmentative communication in work settings and during job interviews (Baker, 1994).

People may have permanent or temporary communication limitations. Groups who typically have permanent limitations include people with physical disabilities: cerebral palsy, head injuries, and degenerative musculoskeletal diseases. At times, however, augmentative communication techniques and devices have assisted people to use their voice even when it was assumed that they may never learn to speak (Light, Beesly & Collier, 1988).

Others may have a temporary loss of communication ability. This group includes people in intensive care units who have been intubated and those who must allow their vocal chords to rest after surgery. The individuals in intensive care units often have immediate needs that they need to communicate. For example, suppose there is a woman whose eyes are swollen shut after an automobile accident. The mascara she had been wearing at the time of the accident was now next to her eye and causing great pain and inflammation. She needs a method to let the nursing staff know the situation with her swollen eyes so that the situation can be handled promptly. Also, an individual may not have been conscious when brought into the hospital. This person needs to ask questions regarding what happened.

These individuals are instructed in using augmentative communication devices to continue communicating. In these situations, the individual can be instructed to squeeze a hand, lift a finger, raise his or her eyebrows, blink, or make any kind of facial gesture when the body part that is in discomfort is mentioned. The alphabet can be recited and the individual can gesture as the desired letter is spoken. Words are spelled out in this fashion. People who are unable to communicate for a period of time and are temporarily paralyzed may find it convenient to use an E-Tran board, discussed in Chapter 5, learn

Morse code, or learn scanning. Scanning can be used with a switch placed next to the forehead with a headband. It is activated by raising the eyebrows. Another switch that works well in this situation is the infrared switch connected to a pair of eyeglasses and activated through an eye blink. Other examples are having boards with the alphabet printed on them kept near the bed. The individual can point to the letters on the board.

The advent of augmentative communication devices and techniques has provided many with more avenues to communicate basic and complex thoughts and ideas to others. Many assistive devices, both low and high technology, are used to improve communication skills. Common devices and systems are discussed here to familiarize the therapist with the technology and terminology. For purposes of organization, communication systems have been divided into written and spoken output. Many occupational therapists have a broader knowledge base in written than spoken communication. Although therapists may not work in the area of AAC where deficits in spoken and written communication are encountered, they will probably work in the area of adapting standard keyboards and recommending alternative keyboards. Therapists should be familiar with alternative keyboards that can be viewed as the next generation of the built-up pencil. Additionally, therapists who have a basic understanding of communication systems are in a better position to relay relevant information to the speech and language pathologist who is also treating the client.

VOCAL AND NONVOCAL OUTPUT— COMMUNICATION SYSTEMS

Although a speech and language pathologist will direct the assessment and choice of augmentative systems, occupational and physical therapists should be familiar with the categories and have a basic understanding of the classifications to assist in the evaluation and training process. AAC systems have four components:

1. Aids and devices—actual physical devices: handheld devices, computers, and dedicated devices
2. Symbol sets—visual or auditory representation of language concepts
3. Communication techniques—methods of transmitting messages: access methods, scanning output
4. Strategies—methods to increase effectiveness of communication: rate enhancements, role playing

Aids and devices have been discussed throughout this book. Some of the commonly used symbol sets are briefly covered in this chapter to help the reader become familiar with them. *Communication techniques* include direct and indirect (scanning); these are addressed in Chapter 3. Role playing strategies are usually the domain of the speech and language pathologist and are not covered here.

There are several communication systems that fall broadly into the categories of unaided and aided systems.

Unaided Systems

Unaided systems familiar to the average person are gestures, vocalizations, and speech. These can be categorized as unaided symbols. Other unaided symbol systems not known to the average individual are the sign languages, for example, American Sign Language, signed English, and key word signing.

Aided Systems

Aided systems include physical, mechanical, and electronic devices that enhance the communication abilities of the individual. Examples of aided systems include adapted keyboards, communication boards, eye-gaze boards, and computers. When the device has the capability of producing speech, it is called a vocal output communication aid.

In aided communication, symbol sets represent language. Symbol sets follow a hierarchy from concrete to abstract. Church and Glennen (1992) have developed a hierarchy that describes this concept (Fig. 7–1). As children develop, they may use several or all of the symbols as outlined here and follow the hierarchy closely. At other times, it is clear that a particular individual is ready for the symbol sets that are more abstract, and these may be the individual's introduction to using symbols to represent language.

Real objects consist of the actual object used as an aid in communication. Real objects are used when the individual needs help to identify the object. A young child or an individual with mental retardation needs the concreteness that a real object provides to understand that a spoken word or picture can represent objects. *Miniature objects* are smaller replicas of the object. They may represent the real object in color and shape. These are used with indi-

Concrete

1. Real Objects

2. Miniature Objects

3. Photographs

4. Line Drawings (color)

5. Line Drawings (black and white)

6. Symbols/Icons

7. Traditional Orthography (written language)

Figure 7–1. Hierarchy of symbol sets representing language. (From Church and Glennen, with permission.)

Abstract

viduals who cannot interpret a photograph or line drawing of an object or with individuals who have limited vision and need the tactile feedback provided by the real or miniature object. Photographs are good quality black and white or color images. They are used to depict objects, verbs, people, places, and activities. Line drawings are a widely used system. A drawing of an object represents a concept about which the individual may wish to talk. The drawings are usually arranged on a communication board by topic. These topics are sometimes color coded to facilitate finding a symbol quickly. For instance, all the food items may be yellow, and all the verbs may be red. Several symbols or icon systems are discussed briefly in the following text. *Orthography* refers to written characters, as in the characters used to print this book. Braille and Morse code fall into this category. Braille is produced through a series of six dots arranged into two columns. Letters are produced by the raised or lowered position of the dot. An individual can use Morse code by pressing one, two, or three switches to produce a series of dots, dashes, or a stop command. The dots and dashes are then translated into symbols recognized by the computer as letters, which can be printed or spoken to the person.

Symbol and Icon Sets

There are several representative symbol sets from which to choose, including photographs, line drawings, and traditional orthography. Various rationales have been used in their development.

Picture Communication Symbols (Fig. 7–2) are a widely used method that provides more than 1800 simple black and white line drawings (Beukelman & Mirenda, 1992), available with or without English labels. The labels are available in 10 different languages (Mayer-Johnson, 1994). Picture Communication Symbols are also available in color and can be obtained on diskettes.

Picsyms (Fig. 7–2) are line drawing symbol sets developed according to a set of defined principles (Carlson, 1985). This system is a combination of predrawn and user-drawn symbols, making the symbols more individually tailored than other symbol sets (ASHA, 1986). Using established principles, new symbols can be generated as needed.

Blissymbolics (Fig. 7–2) were first developed by Charles Bliss (Bliss, 1965) as an international language so people who spoke different languages would have a basis for communication, regardless of their primary language. Shirly McNaughton of Canada began using the abstract symbols as a communication system for people with physical disabilities. She called the communication system Blissymbolics. Blissymbolics has approximately 100 basic symbols that can be used singly or in combination with the other symbols to form vocabulary items.

Minspeak (Fig. 7–3) is an iconic association coding system developed to represent large vocabularies (Baker, Schwartz, & Conti, 1990). The encoding of messages is based on using icons or symbols. Users assign words to

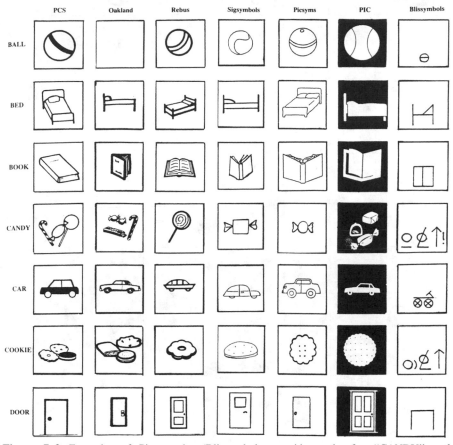

| | PCS | Oakland | Rebus | Sigsymbols | Picsyms | PIC | Blissymbols |

Figure 7–2. Examples of Pictographs (Blissymbols use ideographs for "CANDY" and "COOKIE"). (From ASHA: Augmentative Communication: An Introduction. American Speech-Language-Hearing Association, Rockville, MD, 1986, adapted with permission.)

the symbols that are meaningful to them. Here is an example: The key with a picture of an apple on it could represent food items. The symbol of a truck typically represents travel concepts. However, the truck could also stand for "rig," a slang word for truck, or "rigatoni," a type of pasta. If the user pressed the following keys, apple symbol (for food) and then the truck symbol (for "rig"), the augmentative communication device would say the word "riga-toni." Using this method, several concepts can be stored with a limited number of symbols.

WRITTEN COMMUNICATION

Written communication can involve low to high technology, from paper and pencil to computers and dedicated augmentative communication devices. Each can be individualized. Computers and some dedicated augmentative communication devices have multiple access methods. Additionally, assistive

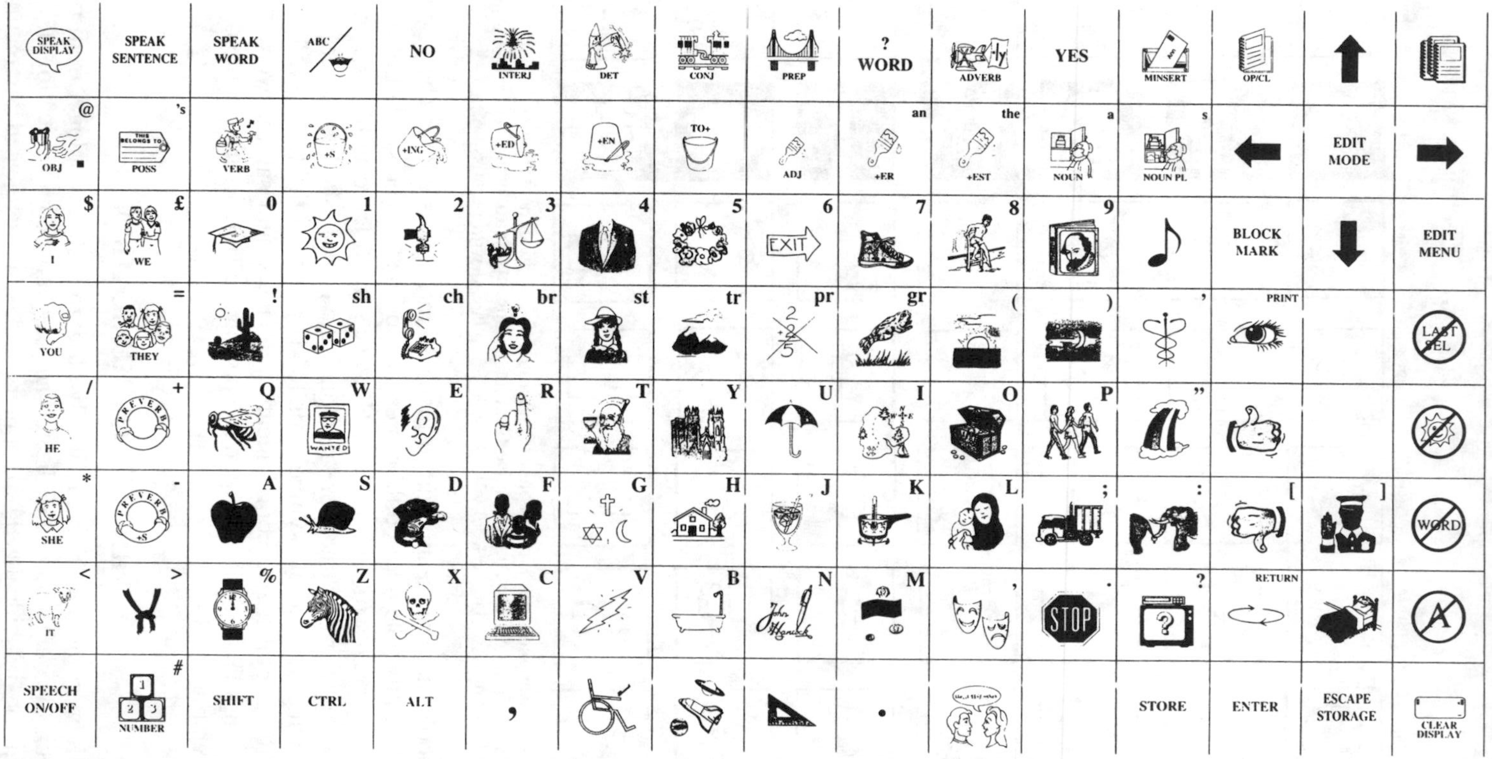

Figure 7-3. Minspeak. (Courtesy of Semantic Compaction Systems, Pittsburgh, PA.)

software can be used with computers to assist in the writing process. Individuals may not be able to use the standard keyboard because of limited range of motion, poor ability to press keys, limited coordination skills, tremors, or excessive movement. When individuals cannot use the standard keyboard, an alternative keyboard may improve the individual's ability to use AT in schoolwork, communication, recreation activities, and other settings. These keyboards have been developed to provide assistance when the standard keyboard is too difficult to use. Various keyboards were developed with specific limitations in mind. Many work with a keyguard. Keyguards are discussed in Chapter 5.

Large Keyboards

Large keyboards have a greater surface area to press for each key. This is helpful for people who find keys on a standard keyboard too small to press accurately. Many of the large keyboards are *membrane* keyboards. A membrane keyboard has a smooth surface. The "keys" do not physically move as do the keys on a standard computer keyboard. The keys on a membrane keyboard are made from electronic switches between conductive membrane layers. Because the membrane layers are thin, a minimal amount of pressure is needed to make the connection.

Features important in membrane keyboards may not be found in other keyboards. Membrane keyboards are programmable. The programming option has obvious benefits: the keyboards can be used as one large switch or different sizes of keys. Typically the smallest size is approximately 1 inch $\times$ 1 inch. These keyboards can also be adjusted for acceptance time. The keyboard can be programmed so that keys must be pressed for a predetermined length of time before the key activates a computer response. This is helpful for individuals who have a tendency to press keys while moving toward the desired key or those who have difficulty releasing the key quickly once they have pressed it.

Here is an example of how this type of keyboard could be used with a child. The keyboard is programmed to act as two large switches for a simple augmentative communication system. The two large switch setup is used to introduce simple choice making, such as being able to tell the teacher whether apple juice or orange juice is desired for a snack. An extension of this example is for the child to use this keyboard to tell the attendant when he or she would like another sip of juice or bite of cookie.

Small Keyboards

Small keyboards are usually recommended for individuals who have limited range of motion and fine coordination. This combination of abilities is frequently seen in neuromuscular diseases. Small keyboards are ideal when the user's range of motion is limited; when he or she cannot reach the keys on the entire keyboard; or when reaching for keys increases fatigue, decreases accuracy, or is too strenuous. Some individuals type with a mouth stick using this kind of keyboard.

Head-Controlled Computer Input Devices

When people are unable to use their arms or legs to press keys on a large or small keyboard, there is an alternative—head pointing. The keyboards used with head pointing systems are not physical pieces of equipment but are virtual keyboards; they exist as an image on the computer screen. Special software is needed to produce the virtual keyboard, but the virtual keyboard works with most software. Users need precise pointing skill with one body part. A pointing device is attached to this body part, typically the head, which is then used to operate the device. A pointing device is attached to the head using a headband, eyeglasses, or cap, or it is adhered to the forehead. The pointing device directs a beam or reflects light to a keyboard presented on the computer screen. Individuals who use these types of keyboards usually have good control over head movement and no or very little control over their limbs. Generally, people with spinal cord injuries are candidates for this type of device.

Keyboard Emulators

An emulator is a device that assists in written and spoken communication by providing several access methods. Keyboard emulators can enhance keyboard entry by slowing down the acceptance rate of keys, changing the key configuration, or changing mouse movements to keyboard strokes. Also, alternative input methods can be connected to the emulator. Examples of alternative input methods include alternative keyboards and switches for scanning or morse code. Frequently software and hardware are involved in the system setup. The first keyboard emulator was the adaptive firmware card for the Apple IIe. Now keyboard emulators are available for the latest computers in Macintosh and personal computer platforms.

A Word About Software

Abbreviation expansion and word prediction software programs are designed to increase typing speed, decrease error rate, and reduce the need to type words and phrases that the typist commonly uses. Abbreviation expansion is now built into some standard word processing software programs. This type of software can also be purchased and integrated with augmentative communication and word processing software. As an abbreviation is typed, the software automatically expands the abbreviation. Here are two examples. The occupational therapist is tired of typing the words "occupational therapy" for every report. To reduce typing, the therapist has programmed the software so that the words "occupational therapy" appear every time the letters "OT" are typed on the keyboard. The word expands every time the two letters are typed. A second example uses initials. An individual who types his or her name for every paper or report can type his or her initials instead, and the name will automatically appear in place of the initials. Abbreviation expansion will work with any combination of letters. Abbreviations that help to remember the words for which they stand usually work best. Some software programs are designed to expand into the word only when a special character is typed after the abbreviation, for instance, the asterisk. Abbreviations must be combinations of letters or symbols that are not commonly used within words, such as "th." This avoids having the expanded word appear in the middle of typing another word.

Word prediction is another method of increasing typing speed, decreasing error rate, and reducing the need to type words and phrases that the typist commonly uses. When the first letter of a word is typed, a box appears on the computer screen that "predicts" what the word might be. There is a number next to each predicted word. Instead of typing the next letter in the word, the typist types in the number. The computer then enters the word onto the screen where the typist was typing. Then the typist continues with the next word. If none of the "predicted" words was the desired word, the typist types the next letter and the software program again "predicts" words that begin with those two letters. Words that the typist uses frequently can be programmed into the word prediction software. Some predicting software programs can "learn," meaning that as the typist continues using this software program, the software will remember the words that the typist uses frequently, and those words will appear in the predicted words list.

Working together, these systems create an environment that increases speed of written or spoken communication. They also decrease typing errors, thereby reducing the need to correct errors. Thus, a well chosen, customized system creates the least amount of fatigue and the greatest degree of efficiency for the user.

Case Study

ANNA

Anna is a 6-year-old girl with significant neurologic impairment due to an episode of hemolytic uremic syndrome 18 months ago. This resulted in neuromuscular incoordination of all voluntary muscles; however, she is able to walk unaided. Anna's speech is partially intelligible for single words, but longer utterances are unintelligible. She has been referred to the augmentative communication clinic to help her find alternative methods for speech and written communication.

Her speech was fairly well understood by family members but not by others, such as teachers and classmates. In context, the family could understand her most of the time; however, if the context was unknown, family members had a difficult time understanding Anna. Her teacher stated that her academic work was at first-grade level. However, she also stated that Anna was slower than the other children in finishing school-work. In part, this was because Anna had difficulty handwriting. Samples of Anna's handwriting were provided by her mother. They were illegible. Anna was referred for an augmentative communication assessment for her written and spoken needs. Devices capable of spoken and written output would need to be evaluated to address all her communication needs.

Speech and Language Assessment

Anna was given several language tests: receptive one-word picture vocabulary, expressive one-word picture vocabulary, test of auditory comprehension language, and clinical evaluation of language fundamentals. Scores from these speech and language tests indicated that Anna's receptive and expressive language was at or above average. However, Anna's spontaneous speech was unintelligible. These test results mean that the speech and language pathologist tested Anna in her vocabulary choices and sentence structure to evaluate if they were age appropriate. The speech and language pathologist asked her questions. As Anna answered, the speech and language pathologist noted the grammar, word endings chosen, and vocabulary. In addition, Anna was tested in her ability to interact—how she started and ended conversations and her ability to take turns during a conversation. Her scores in these areas were above age level. She used the proper grammar, chose vocabulary that was considered above age level, and used complex sentence structures. However, she had difficulty with articulation. For example, the speech and language pathologist could hear that Anna was trying to end a word using past tense, but Anna could not articulate the ending clearly.

Access Assessment

Anna was observed by the occupational therapist for posture and manipulation skills as she sat on the floor and played with a toy. She sat in "W" sitting posture and leaned on one arm for additional support. With her right hand, she played with the toy that had a large latch. She tried unsuccessfully to unlatch the toy first by using her index finger and then by banging it on the floor. In addition, she performed some prehension activities, such as drawing and picking up small objects. These activities were included to form a general idea of her ability to manipulate items she might be asked to use in school and to provide information about dexterity. Anna exhibited low tone throughout her body while engaged in these activities.

During the next part of the evaluation, Anna sat in a child-sized chair with her feet flat on the floor at a child-sized table. Anna was given the Green Dot Test (described in Chapter 3) with different keyboards.

Results of the Access Assessment

The results of the Green Dot Test demonstrated that Anna was able to reach all keys on the Macintosh computer. However, at times she was unable to isolate one key and unintentionally pressed two keys. She knew which key she was supposed to press; however, 50% of the time, her finger slipped off the intended key and pressed the adjacent key. Her average score from the Green Dot Test was 2 errors, 15 seconds.

A keyguard was placed over the standard keyboard to prevent her finger from pressing keys unintentionally. Using this low-technology device, she was able to press the keys accurately. Her average score from this Green Dot Test was no errors, 12 seconds.

Anna found the keyguard awkward to use. She slid her finger into the opening using the edge of the hole as a guide. She complained that this hurt her finger. Using the edge of the hole could become abrasive to the skin on the side of her finger over a long period; therefore, another keyboard was evaluated.

Anna was given the Green Dot Test with a membrane keyboard using a programmed setup for 1-inch keys, The keyboard was inclined approximately 1 inch to help her see and reach the keys. In addition, the response time (the amount of time they needed to be pressed before accepting) was increased. Her average score was no errors, 10 seconds. Anna liked the feel of the keys and commented that they were easy to push.

Recommendations

Recommendations for Anna were the following:

- Participate in speech and language therapy five times a week to improve intelligibility and increase oral-motor control and coordination.
- Use the Macintosh computer connected to an Intellikeys keyboard for schoolwork. (A Macintosh was chosen because it was the type of computer used at her school.)
- Continue occupational therapy to improve coordination skills.

Anna will continue to use her speech with familiar listeners. In the classroom, she will use a combination of speech and an augmentative communication device. Recommendations were to use the Macintosh computer because it was readily available in her classroom and school, Macintalk Pro (intelligible text-to-speech software) as an augmentative communication tool, and the Intellikeys keyboard using the 1-inch keys in place of the standard keyboard for computer access. The Macintosh computer in the classroom is a nonportable system. During recess and lunch time, she will rely totally on speech for communication. In the beginning as Anna is gaining familiarity with all the communication strategies, her teacher will encourage her and her friends to play board games where a predictable and limited vocabulary is needed.

Case Study

SHARON

Sharon is a 53-year-old woman with diabetes, arthritis, and a history of cerebrovascular accident (CVA). Six months ago, while pursuing a master's degree in social work, she suffered a CVA. The CVA left her with severe dysphonia, incoordination of respiration and phonation, and incoordination of articulation consistent with oral-facial dyskinesia. This means that Sharon can form words and can articulate them, but she cannot coordinate a stream of air from her lungs needed to produce sound. Therefore, most of her speech is unintelligible. Facial weakness was noted on the right side with mild to moderate deficits in lip and tongue movements. In addition, she has right-sided weakness.

Sharon came to the augmentative communication clinic using a scooter. She was accompanied to this assessment by her daughter who acted as an interpreter throughout the assessment. She was interested in exploring options available to communicate verbally and in written form. Within 6 months, she will finish her master's degree in social work. At that time, she will begin seeking employment. Therefore, she will definitely need a device to provide assistance in written and verbal communication.

Because of Sharon's medical history of CVA, in addition to other medical conditions, the prognosis that traditional speech therapy could improve her ability to phonate was not strong; therefore, Sharon was referred to an augmentative communication clinic to assess her options. Sharon expressed a keen desire to evaluate augmentative communication devices that would enable her to contribute to class discussions, ask teachers questions, answer the telephone, and write class assignments. In addition, she wanted a device that she could use when interviewing for jobs and in the work setting once she graduated.

Sharon's requirements for a device were that it could be used in face-to-face settings and when making and receiving telephone calls. She also needed to be able to print out messages and speak. In addition, it needed to be easy to manipulate because she was only able to use her right hand for gross movements such as carrying and holding paper securely. She felt that ease of use would be most important because the device needed to fulfill so many roles.

The assessment team agreed that using one system would mean learning the commands for only one device and thus reduce training and possible purchase costs. Moreover, there was not enough funding to purchase two systems, one for home use and one for school use.

Assessment

Sharon's ability to use her hands to access keyboards was evaluated. From watching her maneuver her scooter, sign papers, and straighten her clothing, it seemed apparent that Sharon's fine motor control using her left hand was fully intact. She was asked to type her name and a sentence on a keyboard connected to a computer in the clinic. She made no errors and was able to complete the task easily with her left hand. It was clear that Sharon would be a left-hand typist and would need to practice to obtain this skill but that it would certainly be an attainable goal.

Because of Sharon's dysphonia, the speech and language pathologist on the team reviewed several augmentative communication devices. The device needed to have the following features:

1. A legible screen. Sharon used two sets of glasses, one for seeing objects far away and one for reading. The screen had to be legible so that she could use it to type reports and communicate to others without causing eye strain.
2. Capability of verbal and written communication. The device needed to be versatile so that it could be used as an augmentative communication aid and to produce written documents. Therefore, computers were evaluated because they are able to fulfill both roles easily. Further written output needed to be on standard $8\frac{1}{2} \times 11$-inch paper for assignments, correspondence, and resumes.
3. Speech synthesizer. The synthesizer would replace her voice.
4. A small keyboard. She would be using only the fingers on her left hand to access the device.
5. A system that would accept abbreviations. This would reduce typing words and phrases she used frequently.
6. Portability. Sharon needed to take the device to school and have it secured to her scooter.

The Epson HX-20 Speech Pac with Logical Letter Code and Female "Real Voice" and a notebook computer with speech synthesizer and special software were reviewed. The Epson was reviewed because it has a letter encoding capability and is lightweight. However, it does not have the print-out capability onto 8½ × 11-inch paper. If Sharon used the Epson, she would still need to purchase a second device that had the print-out capability. Therefore, the Epson while a worthwhile device, was unsuitable for Sharon's needs. The second device that was reviewed was a notebook computer. A notebook computer can help Sharon take notes in class, prepare papers for course assignments, function as an augmentative communication device, and run on battery power up to 4 hours. In addition, its screen is larger than the Epson's and is adjustable.

Recommendations

Final recommendations included a desk; portable notebook computer; voice synthesizer; EZ Keys software (by Words+), a word prediction program; a typing program to teach typing skills; a word processing program; an electronic calendar; a 15-inch monitor; and a speaker phone. As the team continued talking with Sharon, it was clear that using her kitchen table and living room couch would not be adequate as places for studying. She needed a place designated for work where she could keep her books, monitor, telephone, and computer. Sharon and her daughter were able to determine the desk size that could be accommodated in the living room. They also discussed furniture rearrangements to accommodate the desk. The computer would be placed on the desk with the keyboard near her left hand. This computer workstation arrangement should prevent back and neck pain from using the computer for prolonged periods. The computer, as previously discussed, will be used as an augmentative communication device and to take notes and write reports. The voice synthesizer plugs into the computer and works with EZ Keys to "speak" what Sharon types. The EZ Keys software prediction program should increase typing speed and decrease errors. The typing program helps Sharon practice using her left hand for typing and pressing the keys quickly instead of having to search for a key letter by letter. The electronic calendar stores phone numbers, meetings, and homework assignments. This helps Sharon organize tasks as she finishes school. When at home, Sharon plugs her 15-inch monitor into the computer and speaker phone. They are kept on the desk where Sharon can easily plug them into her computer when she returns home from school. The 15-inch monitor is used at home when she is writing extensively. The font size is enlarged on the screen, and the monitor placed at the height of her eyes. When Sharon uses the telephone, the computer automatically dials, eliminating the task of dialing.

Under the direction of the occupational therapist, the technician was called in to mount the computer onto the scooter. The therapist demonstrated to the technician how the final placement should look. This was a location where Sharon had no difficulty reaching the keys. The therapist gave the technician a list of requirements that the mounting needed to have: no holes drilled into the computer case because this would void the warranty and possibly damage the computer, a method for securing and removing the computer that Sharon could perform independently, and attaching the mount in a way that does not interfere with driving. With these requirements in mind, the technician fabricated a mounting system from polycarbonate plastic. A ring clamp was used to fasten the mount to the scooter's steering post. The computer slipped into a sleeve, and gravity helped hold the computer in place. Sharon was able to place the computer in the sleeve and remove it easily with one hand.

The occupational therapist worked with Sharon on how to operate her computer using the EZ Keys software and helped her develop a personalized list of abbreviations. The occupational therapist then showed Sharon how to position her computer on the desk so that she would also have forearm support. Forearm support would help prevent fatigue, give her arm stabilization, and possibly reduce typing errors. With the recommendations made, Sharon was able to finish school. She is now in the process of working with the school's placement office to develop her resume and begin searching for a job.

The therapist's role in these two cases is slightly different. With Anna, the therapist's role was to continue therapy to help her develop coordination. In addition, Anna's therapist will periodically review the classroom situation by ensuring that the computer is placed on a table with the screen at eye level and the keyboard is at the height of her hands when her elbows are flexed to 90 degrees with her forearms parallel to the floor. The therapist will also ensure that the chair provides trunk support. For Sharon, the therapist helped her set up the software so that she would be using it to its fullest potential. In Sharon's home, the therapist arranged the furniture to accommodate the desk. With Sharon's input, the therapist placed the monitor and telephone on the desk so that they were convenient to reach and use. These two case studies demonstrate some of the therapist's roles in communication situations.

STUDY QUESTIONS

1. All too frequently young children are not given augmentative communication devices because someone decides that are "not ready."

What characteristics or behaviors would you look for that might indicate "readiness" for consideration of augmentative communication?
2. What aspects of visual perception become critical when considering an augmentative communication device for a child or an adult? Can you think of tools that may be useful in assessing skills in this area when the individual does not have fine motor skills sufficient to allow him or her to draw, write, point, or construct three-dimensional designs?

REFERENCES

ASHA (1986). *Augmentative communication: An introduction.* Rockville, MD: American Speech-Language-Hearing Association.

Baker, B. R. (1994). *Pittsburgh employemnt conference,* Pittsburgh, PA.

Baker, B. R., Schwartz, P. J. & Conti, R. V. (1990). Minspeak models and semantic relationships (pp. 14–15). Seattle WA: Fifth Annual Minspeak Conference Proceedings.

Beukelman, D. R. & Mirenda, P. (1992). *Augmentative and alternative communication, management of severe communication disorders in children and adults.* Baltimore: Paul H. Brooks.

Bliss, C. (1965). *Semantography.* Sydney, Australia: Semantography Publications.

Carlson, F. (1985). Picsyms categorical dictionary. Lawrence, KS: Baggeboda Press.

Church, G. & Glennen, S. (1992). *The handbook of assistive technology.* San Diego: Singular Publishing Group.

Light, J. Beesly, M. & Collier, B. (1988). Transition through multiple augmentative and alternative communication systems: A three-year case study of a head-injured adolescent. *Augmentative and Alternative Communication, 4*(1), 2–14.

Mayer-Johnson Company (1994). *Augmentative communication products.* Solana Beach, CA.

BIBLIOGRAPHY

ASHA (1989). *Competencies for speech-language pathologists providing services in augmentative communication.* Rockville, MD: American Speech-Language-Hearing Association, pp. 107–110.

CHAPTER 8

ENVIRONMENTAL CONTROL UNITS

Assistive Technology Guide

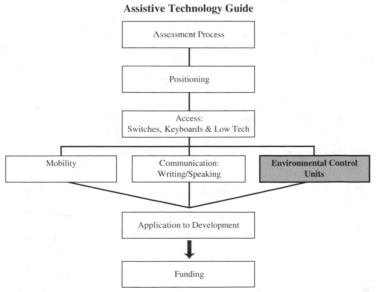

Assessment Process

Positioning

Access:
Switches, Keyboards & Low Tech

Mobility | Communication:
Writing/Speaking | **Environmental Control Units**

Application to Development

Funding

Environmental control units (ECUs) provide a method for people with severe disabilities to operate appliances or devices. The terms environmental control unit, environmental systems, and environmental controls indicate the ability to control one or several electrical appliances or devices. People who use these controls are typically extremely limited physically, such as those with high quadriplegia or muscular degenerative diseases who have very limited range of motion. The goal of using an ECU is to increase the user's independence. Appliances that are commonly connected to ECUs are television sets, videocassette recorders (VCRs), telephones, lights, computers, drapes, and bed controls. ECUs provide the mechanism to accomplish tasks that are otherwise impossible for people with severe disabilities to complete. These include such tasks as manipulating small buttons and dials like the ones found on most appliances. With an ECU, individuals with severely limited motor control can turn on the television or make private telephone calls without the help of a care provider.

ECUs can be found in work, home, and school settings. At work, individuals might use an ECU to place telephone calls. At home, one might use it to change the position of an electric bed, make a telephone call, and turn on the television. At school, an ECU might be used to control a tape recorder for note taking. ECUs range in price from $25 to several thousands of dollars.

ENVIRONMENTAL CONTROL UNIT COMPONENTS

There are three main components to any ECU: the input device, the control unit itself, and the appliance(s) (Fig. 8–1). The *input device* controls the ECU by one of the following: (1) direct selection, such as by using a keypad, keyboard, joystick, or control panel; (2) a set of switches, either single or dual control (see Chapters 4 and 5 for more detail); (3) voice control. The *control unit* itself is the central processing unit, or the "brain" of the device. This is where the input signal is translated into an output signal, and an appliance is given direction. Finally, there is the *appliance*. The appliance can be nearly any electronic equipment. Each of these components is discussed in greater detail in the following sections.

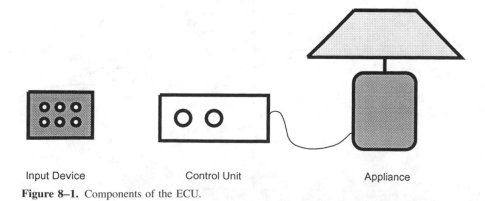

Input Device   Control Unit   Appliance

Figure 8–1. Components of the ECU.

Input Devices

There are several input devices that can make use of whatever voluntary movement the individual has to control the ECU. The common ones are discussed here.

Direct Selection

In the context of ECUs, direct selection involves operating different appliances. Examples of direct selection are a keyboard, such as those used with computers to operate the ECU, or a control panel with buttons. Alternatively, a joystick may be used to activate a different function of an appliance with each direction it is moved.

A computer-controlled ECU can also be a form of direct selection. Computer software programs are available to control appliances. The user progresses through several menus and then presses individual keys to give a command or series of commands to each appliance controlled by the ECU. Typically, people who spend a great deal of time at their computer will choose this option. They prefer to interface with their ECU through their computer rather than find space for an additional input device on their wheelchair or desktop. Alternative computer input methods, such as an optical head pointer, can operate the ECU and the standard keyboard.

Switches

In the simplest arrangement, a single switch activates one appliance, such as a lamp, television set, or radio. Expanding on this simple arrangement, several switches can be used, with each switch controlling a different appliance. When the client has the cognitive capability and desires, one or two switches can be used in a scanning array to operate several appliances and different features of each appliance. The switch is activated, the scanning begins, and the user chooses one of several options. The appliance operations may be in one array, or they may be in a complicated branching system. For example, lights may be in one branch with choices for on, off, and dim; the television and VCR controls are in another branch with choices for on, off, volume control, channel changing, and VCR functions. The order of the items is usually configured so that appliances the individual uses frequently or needs in an emergency are placed at the beginning of the scanning array. Typical setups place emergency telephone numbers early in the array.

Voice Control

Some ECUs can be configured to accept the user's voice as the input method. The ECU can decipher a few words and interpret this into controlling appliances. The user practices speaking key words into a microphone to train the machine to recognize the user's voice. The actual word that is spoken is not essential to operating a voice-controlled system. However, consistency in using the same vocal utterance, voice inflection, and volume level are critical to successfully using this type of ECU input method. Training time and the reliability of the ECU's understanding the user's voice vary. Variability depends on the control unit, fatigue, and the user's ability to make an utterance with the same intonation, volume, and speech pattern.

Control Unit

The control unit contains the wires and circuits where a signal is translated into an actual function, such as turning on the lights. It interprets the signal sent from the input device and activates an appliance.

Appliance

Appliances that are commonly connected to an ECU are those that do not need any other labor for them to work properly. For instance, an ECU would not work connected to a washing machine or vacuum cleaner because those household items need other labor to complete a task. ECUs work well with electric doors, television sets, radios, or lights because no other labor is involved when using them.

CONTROL STRATEGIES

Basically, four control strategies are used to operate ECUs: ultrasound, infrared, radio control, and AC power. Each has advantages and disadvantages. By understanding the differences, therapists can help consumers choose which one will give the best service, depending on individual needs and desires.

Ultrasound

Ultrasound is based on high-frequency sound waves. The sound wave used is above the range of human hearing. A frequency is initiated through the input device, the ultrasound signal reaches the control box, and the control box activates an appliance.

Advantages

The ultrasound waves bounce around the room, and the control box (receiver) detects them. Hence, the user does not have to point the control device directly at the control box. The ultrasound transmitter can be located anywhere in the room and can send signals to the control box located in the same room. The setup is wireless, and the input devices are small and portable.

Disadvantage

The transmitter must be in the same room as the control box. The user cannot control an appliance in one room while physically operating the ECU from another room.

Infrared

Infrared pulses are initiated by the user from the remote control and transmitted to the control box. The control box sends the signal to the appropriate appliance. This is the type used in VCR remote controllers commonly found in homes today.

Advantage

The input devices are portable. This means that they can be mounted to a wheelchair and can be used from different locations within the room.

Disadvantage

The user must point the input device directly at the control box or the receiver. If something is between the input device and the control box, the signal cannot be transmitted to the control box. For example, if a person tries to change the channel on the television set using the remote control, and an object, an individual, or a piece of furniture is in between the remote control and the receiver, the signal cannot reach the control box. People using this device from a wheelchair may have difficulty lining up the remote controller and the control box. If a child leaves a toy that covers the receiver, the user will be unable to use the ECU until the toy is removed.

Radio Control

Radio control frequencies are the same radio waves used in the radios found in homes and cars. They are also used in toys, baby monitors, and garage door openers. Radio control technology uses radio frequencies to transmit control codes to appliances.

Advantages

Radio transmission is not blocked by objects between the input device and the control box. Therefore, the user can be in one room and signal an appliance in another room. Additional wiring is not necessary to install this type of ECU.

Disadvantage

The radio frequencies are limited in the distance they can travel. The average range is 50 to 200 ft. If the input is more than 200 ft. from the control box, it probably will not activate the appliance. Interference from another control unit is possible. Appliances can be activated when the user does not press his or her switch. For instance, when neighbors open their garage door with a radio frequency device, the person using an ECU could have a light turned on.

AC Power

AC power uses the existing electrical wiring in the dwelling to send signals that will activate appliances. The input device is either part of the control box or a remote unit. The control box is plugged into the wall. The appliances are plugged into an appliance module that is plugged into an electrical outlet.

Advantages

Existing house wiring is used; therefore no wiring installation is needed.

Disadvantages

The control box and appliance modules must be programmed. Each appliance module has two dials. The dials allow the appliance module to be programmed for each appliance. Several electrical outlets are needed. Older homes that have older electrical wiring can be problematic.

ASSESSMENT GUIDELINES

Before recommending ECUs, several issues need to be addressed. If an ECU is provided without first addressing these issues, there is a greater chance that it will not meet the user's needs. The user may remain dependent on someone else to perform the activity. The funding available for such devices may be depleted. To prevent this type of unfortunate incident from occurring, it is best to have an evaluation session to answer the questions posed below and allow the user to try out several devices before a final recommendation is made. If ECUs are not on hand, it is possible to have vendors lend them so that the appropriate device can be selected. This helps to ensure that the user understands what types of tasks the device can and cannot perform. An evaluation that includes an actual trial with the device can make the therapist's letter of justification stronger. The letter can describe the client's actual success controlling the ECU.

Additionally, the therapist must understand the tasks ECUs can and cannot perform. As the therapist gathers information from the potential user, he or she can begin to eliminate ECUs that would not be suitable for the individual. Also, as the therapist and individual discuss the user's needs and goals, the therapist can provide a clearer picture of available options.

The issues, presented as questions, follow.

What Does the User Want the ECU to Do?

The therapist should ask the user what tasks he or she expects to be able to accomplish by using an ECU. This tells the therapist if the potential user understands the function ECUs can provide. Second, this tells the therapist what functions the user wants from an ECU.

What Are the User's Functional Capabilities?

What input devices should the user try to operate with an ECU? The reader should refer to Chapters 3 and 4 on access and switches for more information on access assessments. Therapists should know what access methods are available to the user. For instance, can the user apply a direct selection technique to a small area using a mouth stick or finger? Is he or she able to press a switch with his or her knee? Some ECUs are voice activated and need no physical input. As noted in Chapter 4, the input devices the client can best control should be examined. The input device selected needs to be matched to the ECU that can handle this type of input. Some ECUs allow for several input options. The therapist should know which ECU works with the type of input the client can control.

What Type of Feedback Does the User Need?

Controllers usually provide visual or auditory feedback. Knowing the environment in which the user will control the ECU will help to determine the type of feedback that will be most appropriate. If the user is in an office with many workers, auditory feedback might bother other people, or the environment might be too noisy to make use of auditory feedback. In another situation, the user would not want auditory feedback to disturb others, such as in a library or classroom lecture. In this case, an ECU with visual feedback may be more appropriate. In addition, characteristics of the individual will help determine this issue. If the user has a hearing loss, auditory feedback may be inappropriate. Thus, when determining "best" feedback from the ECU to the user, more than one aspect of use must be considered.

Where Will the ECU Be Used?

Does the user need the ECU at home, work, school, or other environments? Will it be used in just one setting, or does it need to be used in several settings? Can more than one ECU be purchased? Must they be the same? Perhaps the needs are different in the different environments; therefore, one type of system can be used in one location and a different system in another location. A computer may be used across all environments, but it may be necessary to control lights and answer the telephone at home and at the office. The type of ECU chosen will depend on how flexible it must be.

Will the ECU Be Used in One or Several Rooms?

Some ECUs allow the user to move from room to room; others can operate only in one room. Knowing the number of rooms in which the ECU is to be used helps determine the type of ECU that should be recommended.

How Much Space Does the ECU Require?

Once the rooms where the ECU will be used have been determined, the therapist should know approximately how much space is available in the rooms in which the equipment will be placed and note the approximate size of the equipment needed. Taking room measurements at this stage avoids costly mistakes later as the equipment is being installed.

What Is the User's Cognitive Status?

Although the therapist may not administer a cognitive assessment, he or she should have a general knowledge of the user's cognitive capabilities. If the user has limited cognitive abilities, then the recommended ECU should not require extensive training, setup, or programming. A direct link that is easy to use will be a good fit between the user and the ECU. An example is a system that uses colored switches. Each colored switch operates a different device. A sticker the same color as the switch can be placed on the device. This color coding assists the user in remembering which switch operates which device. In addition, the therapist should understand the complexity of the ECU he or she is considering recommending. The ECU should not be overwhelming or cognitively demanding for the user. If the ECU assessment is a portion of a total assessment, the therapist may already have a good grasp of the user's cognitive abilities.

What Positions Will the User Be Taking?

The therapist should determine if the user spends most of his or her time in the wheelchair, lounge chair, or bed or in different places. Many times, an ECU will be usable from a wheelchair because the user was evaluated in his or her wheelchair in the clinic; however, later it is discovered that at home, the user spends the majority of time in bed. Discovering this information after the recommendation has been made can mean requiring additional work and reassessment, retrofitting the input device, or requesting additional funding to purchase a second input device that can be controlled from the bed.

Who Can Repair the Equipment?

It is important to have someone assume the responsibility of making simple repairs and performing troubleshooting tasks. Sometimes this person emerges as the one in the family who is attracted to gadgetry and fixes everything in the home anyway. At other times, someone needs to be appointed to complete the setup once the equipment arrives and maintain it once it is in use.

Is Funding Available?

Knowing the user's price range will help narrow the choices of which ECUs the user should try out. In some instances, price should not be considered; the functional capability and the user's needs should be put first. If, however, the user is paying for the ECU, then price needs to be discussed before the user tries devices that he or she cannot afford.

Does the User Need Portability?

Some ECUs work in one room only, and some can be set up to control appliances in several different rooms in the dwelling.

The ECU products need to be reviewed to make a good match between user and device. The therapist who has a good grasp of the products will be in a better position to make a recommendation that will satisfy the user.

How Difficult Is the ECU to Install?

The therapist will want to know if additional wiring is needed and the amount of programming and setup required to make the unit operational. Some ECUs can be plugged into wall sockets and installed within a few minutes. Others require wiring skills or need computer software for installation.

Training

Some ECUs are simple systems. The user requires only a minimal amount of training. For other ECU systems, the user requires several hours of training before he or she begins to feel comfortable with it. The therapist needs to make arrangements so that training can be provided. Ideally, the training should occur where the device will be used.

Case Study

LARRY

Larry, a 6-year-old boy, was diagnosed with a head injury after he collided with a car while running across the street. Because of the injury, he has minimal control over all his limbs. His parents want him to be able to participate in some of the leisure activities he pursued prior to the injury so that they can begin to feel they have their "old Larry" back. Before the injury, Larry had enjoyed arcade-type computer games and baking cookies with his mother.

Assessment

An access assessment was performed using the 1- and 2-inch grids suggested by Goosens' & Crain (1992). This assessment was not timed, but observations were used in evaluating Larry's ability to indicate a 1-inch square. During the observations, Larry's hand moved over several squares, and it was difficult for him to localize and stabilize a finger over just one square. Therefore, the 2-inch square grid was used. Larry continued to have difficulty indicating selections that were 2 inches in diameter because of erratic hand and finger movements. Therefore, using switches was indicated. He could easily locate two jelly bean switches if they were placed on his left side and were 3 inches apart.

An arcade-like pinball game software program was found that intrigued Larry. It was set up so that Larry could turn on the computer with a switch connected to a power strip. Larry's father set up the computer so that when it was turned on, it automatically started the pinball game for Larry. Instead of the dual jelly bean setup noted previously, an alternative keyboard was considered because of its versatility. The pinball game needed two keypresses to play the game. Intellikeys keyboard was programmed to act like two large switches. The Intellikeys keyboard is an enlarged membrane keyboard. Keys can be programmed to be any size. The right half of the keyboard was the first switch, and the left half was the second switch. This keyboard was recommended because of its ability to meet future needs. If Larry's motor skills improved and he was able to accurately press keys using a large keyboard, this equipment could be reprogrammed from two-switch emulation to a keyboard with large keys. This eliminates the need of purchasing new equipment as Larry's needs change. His parents hoped that later Larry could use this keyboard for more academic computer applications as his needs changed.

Having determined appropriate input for Larry, the Powerlink 2 Control Unit was chosen. The Powerlink 2 is a simple ECU. It controls two appliances with two switches. In the home, Larry's mother plugged her electric mixed (pedestal model) and the jelly bean switch into the Powerlink 2. Once all the ingredients were in the mixer, Larry could do the mixing. At Christmas, they realized that Larry was no longer able to help with trimming the Christmas tree. He could light the Christmas tree lights with a Powerlink 2 Control Unit. During the tree trimming, the lights and the jelly bean switch were plugged into the Powerlink 2 Control Unit. A small table was placed by the tree so that the jelly bean switch was easily available. It was Larry's daily job to turn the Christmas tree lights on and off.

Larry's parents purchased the Intellikeys keyboard and the Powerlink 2 Control Unit to provide independence. They also hoped that the flexibility of these two devices would provide for increased independence for some years to come. In the future, they want to look into ECUs that will allow greater independence for Larry, such as making telephone calls.

Larry's parents are always looking for new ways to include their son in daily family activities. They want him to have job responsibilities appropriate to his age. By teaching him how to perform chores that are appropriate to his age now, they hope that he will grow into a responsible adult who can take on adult responsibilities. He should be able to do this with the assistance of ECUs.

Case Study

LINDA

Linda is a 53-year-old married woman with amyotrophic lateral sclerosis. She referred herself to the clinic for an augmentative communication device and information on other devices that might help her continue to complete tasks independently. She is experiencing increased fatigue due to the disease process and some weakness in her left arm, leg, and the musculature of her face. She wants to avoid depending on her husband and daughter for all tasks.

At the time of the first assessment, Linda was walking with a cane for short distances but could not speak. She indicated that she found vocalizing frustrating and exhausting. She was using an erasable pad and marker to communicate. Linda could type using a computer keyboard and dial the telephone independently. However, she had no method for communicating over the phone. Her three main goals were to continue being an active communicator face to face, to use the telephone to maintain contact with friends and her daughter who attends college out of town, and to operate the lights and television. Providing services to Linda and accomplishing these three goals came in a series. The face-to-face communication goal was considered first, keeping the other two goals in mind and ensuring that all the equipment was compatible. She was provided with a notebook computer with AAC software and a voice synthesizer. As the first goal of active communication was resolved, the other two goals could be more carefully evaluated. Linda was shown an ECU device that she could activate from her computer. It would enable her to use the telephone and television from her bedroom and family room provided she could carry the computer to the different locations.

When reviewing possible combinations of equipment for Linda, it was important to keep in mind that her ability to control input methods would change as her muscle control deteriorated. Therefore, systems that had multiple input strategies built into the system were closely reviewed. These were considered a better investment than buying one system that met her present needs but would need to be replaced as Linda's needs changed. Although currently she had enough muscle control to use a keyboard, the disease would continue to decrease her ability.

At the time of the evaluation, she could type using a hunt and peck method with the index finger of her right hand. She could open the computer and turn it on independently. She could perform some fine motor manipulation tasks that did not require strength. For many daily tasks she performed in her home, she was able to accomplish the manipulation involved, but she was unable to travel to the input device, such as turning on the television or light. It was more convenient and conserved her energy to remain seated and control her environment from one location.

After reviewing all the possible options, Words+ EZ Keys and U-Control ECU equipment were recommended. The ECU and augmentative communication device work through a notebook computer. Input methods and software could be changed as Linda's needs changed. Separate software that would dial the telephone and allow her to use her augmentative communication software with a speaker phone was also recommended.

The U-Control is an ECU that uses an infrared control strategy. The controller plugs into Linda's notebook computer. The software for the augmentative communication system was also installed on the computer's hard disk. She operated the lights and television through the U-Control, and when she could no longer use the keyboard, she would be able to use the Scanning WSKE; the single switch, scanning input method. This ECU could be used directly with her augmentative communication software so she could independently use the telephone. Scanning WSKE interfaced in a similar manner as EZ Keys; therefore, Linda maintained her ability to control the lights and television set with the U-Control. When Linda was still active, her family carried the U-Control and her notebook computer to the kitchen and plugged it into the telephone. From there she could use the phone and did not need any other assistance. At the end of the day, her family returned the equipment to her bedroom and plugged it in so she could prepare for bed and use the phone and television set from her bed.

Once her disability no longer allowed her to use the keyboard on her portable computer, she began using Scanning WSKE. She was still able to use the phone, the ECU, and her augmentative communication device. In this way, she remained an active telephone user. She was able to call her mother once a day and her husband could call her from work. Linda was satisfied with the ECU. She felt that it gave her a level of independence that she could not have realized without it.

STUDY QUESTIONS

1. Combining your prior knowledge and experience with the information on types of ECUs presented in this chapter, design a table listing the pros and cons of each, and brainstorm the client needs that might lead you to choose one over the other.

Don't Use It If ...	Cons	Type of ECU	Pros	Use It If ...
the room is crowded and there is a high likelihood that things will get in the way	it must be aimed directly at the receiver to activate the device	Infrared	portable, can be attached to wheelchair	the user wants to be able to use the ECU from any place in a room, and can aim it at the receiver easily

2. Consider the impact home environment may have on your choices of ECUs for an individual. How would your choice be influenced if you were working with an adult in a group home? A nursing home? An independent apartment?

REFERENCES

Goosens' C. & Crain, S. (1992). Utilizing switch interfaces with children who are severely physically challenged. Austin, TX: Pro-ed.

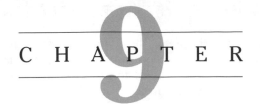

CHAPTER 9

CAN AND SHOULD TECHNOLOGY BE USED AS A TOOL FOR EARLY INTERVENTION?

Shelly J. Lane, PhD, OTR, FAOTA, and
Susan G. Mistrett, MS, Ed

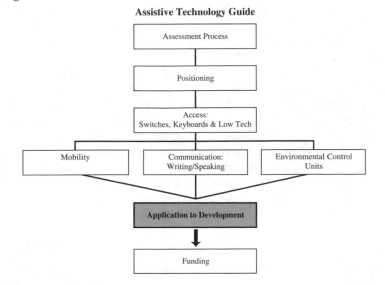

Assistive Technology Guide

Assessment Process

Positioning

Access:
Switches, Keyboards & Low Tech

Mobility | Communication:
Writing/Speaking | Environmental Control
Units

Application to Development

Funding

The preceding chapters of this book focus on the application of technology to children roughly preschool age to adulthood. The authors have indicated that technology can be used to properly position a child, provide mobility, and give a child access to toys, communication devices, and computers. The point has been made that providing technology to individuals in this age range is not merely a feasible goal, it is crucial to the promotion of optimal development of play, learning, and communication skills. Should technology be offered at even younger ages? Is it an appropriate addition to intervention ideas for the child with disabilities, beginning from birth? Consider the following:

☐ SCENARIO I: ANNA

Anna is 10 months old. She is just beginning to vocalize, is very visually alert, and can reach out to bat at toys when she is on her back. However, Anna has spina bifida and cannot sit independently. Although she has use of her arms, she has some muscle weakness, making it difficult for her to hold and manipulate toys in an age-appropriate manner. For instance, Anna is not able to grasp and hold a toy in one hand unless the toy is very soft, and she has difficulty with other age-appropriate tasks, such as holding two toys simultaneously and banging toys. Anna is not ready to be mobile within her environment, and as such, she is not exploring. Her sound production is limited, and although the sounds capture her mother's attention, they are not used to communicate preferences to her mother. In short, her disability has resulted in several barriers to age-appropriate interaction with toys and people in her environment.

Anna is experiencing difficulty with activities in which typically developing children naturally engage. During the time when typically developing children are learning that their actions produce a response from the people and things in their environment, Anna is learning that she cannot have an impact on her environment. Anna is learning that her muscles are not strong enough to make a toy work, that she cannot sit up and look around, cannot get to the cupboard to find out what is inside, and cannot tell her mother that she would like to have a particular toy. Would the use of some assistive devices give Anna greater freedom within her environment? Could devices be chosen that would be age appropriate, that would be acceptable to Anna's mother, that would help address the needs that Anna's mother sees as priorities for Anna, and that would optimize development for Anna? Logic tells us that the answer to each of these questions is "yes," and this answer is gaining some support from research in the field.

USE OF TECHNOLOGY FOR THE VERY YOUNG CHILD

Between birth and 3 years, children play. Play for typical children has the characteristics of intrinsic motivation and internal control. It is done just because it is fun. Learning takes place vicariously through play, along with development in all major realms—sensorimotor, communication, social-emotional, and cognition (Athey, 1988; Curry & Bergen, 1988; Kaplan-Sanoff, Brewster, Stillwell & Bergen, 1988). This is a time when major changes in skill in all areas of development occur. The child with a disability that interferes with play, and therefore with development in all realms, is at a serious disadvantage. The child may find it difficult or impossible to interact with toys and playmates and may be unable to exert control over the physical and social environment due to physical, cognitive, sensory, or communication barriers. It is highly likely that further development in all areas will be adversely influenced by these barriers to play (Brinker & Lewis, 1982; Bradley, 1985).

Even when these very young children are offered toys and playthings, the situation may not improve for them. Bradley (1985) suggests that although toys and play have the potential to have a strong and positive impact on social and cognitive development, frustration can ensue when toys are too difficult to operate, as they may be for children with disabilities. Similarly, frustration may develop for a child when he or she is improperly positioned for toy access and activation or when the toy is improperly positioned. The absence of toys over which the child can exert control may mean that the child cannot play. Toys then can become an obstacle to learning or objects of frustration, rather than facilitators of the developmental process.

The long-term effects of this "play deprivation" negatively impact the child's motivation to continue the attempt at interaction and environmental control. Jennings, Connors, Stegman, Sankaranarayan, and Medolsohn (1985) report that children with disabilities display less persistence and curiosity than do their peers without disabilities. Reports indicate that the play of children with disabilities differs from that of their nondisabled peers in that play repertoires are more limited, and play is less frequent (Li, 1981; Kaplan & Kopp, 1983). Children with physical disabilities experience real limitations to play, and their play has been described as more often solitary, with less frequent play incidences (Jennings et al., 1985; Bergen, 1991). As reported by parents of children with multiple disabilities, Florey (1971) presented characteristics of play as sedentary and passive, with a limited availability of materials, overemphasis on either large or small motor actions, and parent expectations that were too high or too low. Furthermore, these children may develop learning deficits that complicate the disabilities they are already experiencing. Children with disabilities have been noted to develop a sense of helplessness and incompetence as a result of their inability to control and communicate with the environment. Mastery motivation, a drive to have successful interaction with the physical and social world, is not developed as the child learns what he or she cannot do rather than what he or she can do (Jennings et al., 1985). Such learned helplessness may lead to indifference and apathy in children as young as 2 years old (vanTatenhove, 1987). It is essential that methods be identified that can augment existing play abilities or compensate for limitations imposed by disabilities to avoid these pitfalls in the growth process in infants and children with disabilities.

The Potential of Assistive Technology to Facilitate Play and Development

Assistive technology (AT) applications have been reported to extend the play repertoires and play interactivity of some infants and toddlers with disabilities (Behrmann, 1984; Swinth, Anson, & Deitz, 1993; Brinker & Lewis, 1982; Wright & Nomura, 1985). That is, the very early use of adaptive toys, switches, computers, and powered mobility can be effective in forestalling the development of learned helplessness and learning deficits (Behrmann, & Lahm, 1984; Hanson & Hanline, 1985; Robinson, 1986; vanTatenhove, 1987; Butler, 1988; Douglas, Reeson, & Ryan, 1988; Behrmann, Jones, & Wilds, 1989; Langley, 1990; Bradley, 1994) and may lay the foundation for transition to the use of other needed adaptive devices, such as computers and augmentative communication devices (Williams & Matesi, 1988; Wilds, 1989). In fact, AT may be the *only* way some children with significant disabilities can engage in a physically and socially responsive environment. Technology can put the environment within reach of the child and make it possible for the child to act on and receive a response from the environment (Wilds, 1989). Responsivity of the play environment has also been positively linked with development (Wachs & Gruen, 1982). Thus, AT has the potential to extend the play abilities of very young children with significant disabilities.

Research using AT with infants and young children has primarily emphasized the applications of computers and other "high-tech" technology, for example, powered mobility and augmentative communication devices (Behrmann, 1984; Butler, 1986), to this population rather than examining options of "low-tech" technology (adding switches for toy activation). For the young child, low-tech goes beyond the adaptations defined in Chapter 5. Low-tech adaptations are differentiated here from high-tech devices by cost factors, electronic complexity, training and setup time required, and estimated length of durability and use. Examples of low-tech devices for young children can be found in Table 9–1. While high-tech solutions are sometimes effective for young children (vanTatenhove, 1987; Douglas, Reeson, and Ryan, 1988), some parents may not be ready for this, and some children may reap greater benefits from low-tech options (Warren & Horn, 1987; see Table 9–1).

The use of low-tech AT must be decided on a case-by-case basis. When the child is very young, the therapist must begin with the examination of parental goals, as specified by Public Law 99-457. The law mandates that services from the birth to 3 years must be family focused (Gallagher, Trohanis, & Clifford, 1989). Along with the primary caregiver, service providers can work to define the abilities and needs of a child and from there, identify solutions that can decrease or eliminate the barriers to independent function (Williams, Briggs, & Williams, 1979). The process for the older child differs

Table 9–1. "LOW-TECH" ASSISTIVE TECHNOLOGY

Assistive technology opens up new opportunities for infants and toddlers with disabilities, their families, and caregivers. It can help these children play and participate more fully in home, school, and community settings.

Low-tech assistive technology for play and participation includes aids that do the following:

- Make things easier to turn on (adaptive switch or larger knob)
- Help with seating or offer alternative play positions (swing or chair inserts, Boppy pillows, trays)
- Help a child play (switch toys or switches, extenders on toy parts)
- Help a child communicate (tape recorders and loop tapes, choice boards)
- Help a child to hear or see better (magnifiers, penlights)
- Hold things steady or in place (Velcro or clamps)
- Help a child to be bathed, dressed, or fed (bath supports, built-up utensils)
- Help a child with early learning (picture and storybook software)
- Help a child move (scooters, walkers, push carts)
- Help a child control things (call systems, remote)

somewhat in that the school-aged child may play a more integral role and the family a somewhat less dominant role in determining barriers to learning, play, and environmental interaction and control and in identifying potential solutions to these barriers (NICHY News Digest, 1991).

As low-tech and high-tech options for young children are summarized in the following text, it is important to keep in mind that AT interventions are not an end in and of themselves. Investigators in this field caution that switches and adaptations for toys must be used as the means to a bigger end, that of developing functional skills and independence (Langley, 1990). Setting a child up with an electronic toy and switch and watching the child have an impact on the environment is worthwhile only in that it leads later to choice making, communication, interaction, and development in other domains.

SEATING AND POSITIONING

In Chapter 2, the importance of proper seating as a part of intervention for the child with significant neuromotor disabilities is addressed. Do the same concepts apply to the child in the birth to 3-year-old age range? Clinical experience suggests that other aspects of proper positioning and variations in positioning to promote play and environmental interaction are at least of equal importance. Keeping in mind that the primary role of the child in the birth to 3-year age range is to play, what positions are important? Observation of a typical child at play shows that this child will use his or her available repertoire of positioning options repeatedly throughout a play period. Thus, a typical 10-month-old child may lie prone, supine, roll, sit, assume "all fours," creep, sit, and lie supine again, all in 5 minutes. A 3-year-old child, with a wider repertoire of positioning options, will move in and out of squatting, lying prone to reach under the table for a toy, move back to sitting, and then up to stance. In addition, once mobility is realized, children will run, walk, creep and walk backward at will. Typically, developing young children are often not still! The child from birth until at least 2 years is considered to be in a "sensorimotor" play stage, which means that often movement and position alone are the play activities. This is important to consider when working with the very young child with disabilities that prevent position changes and mobility from developing optimally. Recall Anna, described at the beginning of this chapter. She is not yet mobile, and she is not exploring her environment. She is not able to change positions readily, her body is not overcoming the influence of gravity, and she is not able to move in and out of various positions. Giving Anna mobility would be an appropriate intervention even at her young age.

Another point of consideration in this area is the caregiver, the parent. When the child is very young, a parent may not be ready for a complex seating system, which may seem too cumbersome and too indicative of "disability." The use of low-tech positioning adaptations to provide positioning options may be more acceptable and more useful to parent and child. For instance, adding a seat insert to a stroller, rather than recommending a wheelchair, may serve the needs of the child and the parent and may be more maneuverable within a small home. The choice of adaptations and positioning options should be based on the parent's needs and goals for the child, and the child's current motor skills, needs, and preferences.

Following are some ideas and options for using low-tech adaptations in positioning, with the goal being to enable the child to play. This is not intended to be an exhaustive list, and many therapists may find nothing earth shattering about the ideas. The uniqueness of these ideas may come from thinking of them as low-tech AT designed to promote development and play and thinking of each as one of several options designed to give the child or parent some choices about play position.

Supine

Many children spend a great deal of time supine, and adaptations may not be needed. Our clinical experience indicates that often the supine position may not be optimal because the child may be unable to fight gravity to reach for toys. Using a round pillow, snow or inner tube, or a Boppy (a "U"-shaped pillow), will prevent the neck and trunk overextension commonly seen when children are supine on the floor or bed (Fig. 9–1). This positioning device brings the shoulders forward and the neck into some flexion and can move the child from a flat supine position to a semireclined position. A similar position can be achieved with a small child if he or she is placed in the "well" formed by parental legs in a tailor sit position. Both of these options allow the *en face* position for parent and child and promote cue reading and communication. This position may facilitate the development of reaching from supine to touch the parent's face or hands or bat at toys that are appro-

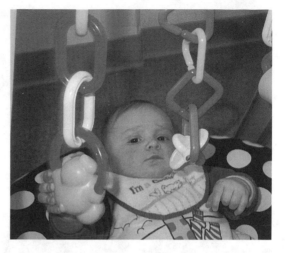

Figure 9–1. Laying supine in a Boppy gives this child head support and brings the shoulders forward, enabling him to reach for and grasp an overhead toy.

priately positioned within the child's overhead reach and visual field. Many types of baby gyms can be used in supine to promote reach, bat, look, and even grasp. Some of these toys allow exchange of the objects that are suspended from them to offer the child many options of interest. They may also offer the therapist and the parent the option of using links to lower the hanging toy to the proper height. Other gyms offer the option of tilt to different angles. The interested parent and therapist will need to explore these options and decide which is best suited to the individual child.

Prone

Prone is a stressful, hard-work position, and many children do not enjoy playing in it. While therapists often tell parents that this position is very important to the development of back and neck muscles and may promote increased strength in the shoulders and arms, if the child cries in this position, the parent is unlikely to use it for play. Therapists may want to begin introducing a child to the prone position by using a therapy ball. Even if the child has difficulty lifting his or her head in prone position, the ball lifts the child from the floor, and in this position the child can still see what is going on in the immediate environment. The addition of a mirror or close-by table outfitted with an appropriate toy may make this initial attempt at prone "play" instead of "work." For children with some degree of head control, the simple addition of a rolled towel or commercially available half-roll or full-roll placed under the arms will give enough support that prone position will be an option for play (Fig. 9–2). For others, using a wedge may help to alleviate some of the stress on the upper trunk; inclining the wedge to bring the child into a more upright position may also be more acceptable to the child. Another alternative is to place the child prone over the parent's lap, with the parent sitting comfortably on the floor or a couch. If the child can impose

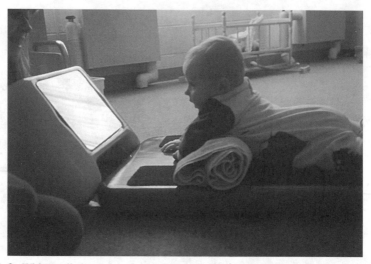

Figure 9–2. With a rolled towel under his arms, Alex's arms are brought forward and his chest is supported. He can now watch himself in the mirror.

movement on this otherwise stationary position, it may become more inter-esting, functional, and fun. Using a small bolster or roll instead of the parent's leg, towel, or wedge may add some degree of mobility to the prone position. Prone positioning over a roll allows the child the option of back and forth movement, and the movement may activate the neck extensors, leading to improved head control in this position. This is an interesting idea because typical children move a great deal. Rarely do they use prone position as a static position for any length of time.

The real key to making this a functional position is to make it fun. If the child cannot lift his or her head to look around or find a toy, mirror, or interesting person in the environment, *it is not fun*, and the child is unlikely to have much tolerance for the position. However, if sufficient head control is present to raise the head, if mobility is present, and if a sufficiently inter-esting toy or person is offered, play in prone position becomes a possibility. Siblings, parents, and other relatives may all provide motivation for the child to lift his or her head with sounds, words, and motions. Mirrors work for some children, because they enjoy viewing their face. Children are attracted to toys that are responsive. Thus, consider a toy that can be activated by the child or caregiver to provide the type of sensory input the child enjoys. For some children, the therapist may need to identify a toy with high stimulus value, that is, with bright lights, loud sounds, or both. For other children, this may be overstimulating, so the parent or therapist must look for toys that are responsive in a more subtle way. The key is to use toys that are appropriately matched to the child's sensory interest *and toys that the child can activate*. When a child's motor skills are limited by disability, battery-operated toys attached to an appropriate switch (a switch the child can successfully activate) may be the ideal solution. Placing Anna on a 1.5-inch wedge, with a jelly-bean switch attached to a battery-operated horse worked to keep her in prone position for about 3 minutes. She was able to activate the switch and lift her head to watch as the horse galloped toward her and then stopped to neigh.

When the child fatigues in prone position, it is time to change positions. Pushing a child to remain in prone position once fatigue sets in is not productive; fatigue will create sloppy and possibly inappropriate positioning, and the child will resist the position in the future, knowing that he or she will be required to maintain it longer than desired. Typical children do not remain in a single position for long periods of time. When they get tired of the position, they move. This same concept must be applied to the child with a disability.

Sidelying

This is another positioning option to consider. Although most children do not use sidelying extensively during play and leisure, it is an available option and should be considered for children with disabilities. The sidelying position has the potential to capitalize on the child's functional skills because it removes gravity from upper extremity reach-like movements, allowing greater freedom of movement for this activity. In addition, gravity actually brings the arms and legs toward midline, which can help the child to be more relaxed (Diamant, 1992). It can be made functional with support to assist in maintaining the position. This support can be from the therapist's or parent's leg or something like a large towel roll. One way to use sidelying is to position the child with his or her head on a pillow. The bottom arm should be brought forward, so that it is out in front of the child. The bottom hip and knee can be kept straight, which may help the child maintain this position, or they may be flexed to match the position of the top hip and knee (Diamant, 1992). The top hip and knee should be slightly flexed, the head placed on a very low pillow or small towel, and the neck at neutral or positioned with some flexion (Fig. 9–3). With the neck in this position, the eyes look directly at the hands and arms, which provides the child with an opportunity to watch his or her hands work and play. A variation on this position is to have the child semi-reclined in the sidelying position. The child is placed between the legs of an adult, and the child's trunk (and head if necessary) are supported and elevated slightly. This position frees up the bottom arm and the top arm to allow for bilateral reach, grasp, and play (Fig. 9–4). Adding an interesting toy or person to this scenario may encourage the child to reach out with the top arm toward the person or toy. The parent can be encouraged to guide the reaching hand toward the object of interest and assist in manipulation or activation if the object used lends itself to this. If the toy is easily activated (i.e., an easy pop-up toy), the child can receive positive feedback for his or her efforts. The therapist or parent should be careful not to use toys that will quickly move

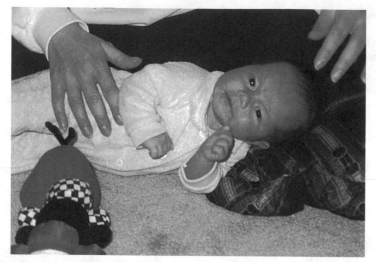

Figure 9–3. Sidelying with a pillow to support the head allows this baby to use both arms for play.

out of reach, because this is not a position that promotes mobility. Not unlike other positions, this one will work only as long as the child remains interested in what is happening in the visual environment he or she can see.

Sitting

For children with some head control but in need of additional trunk support, make sitting functional by exploring options such as a "U"-shaped pillow (i.e., the Boppy) or pillows placed around the child to provide some

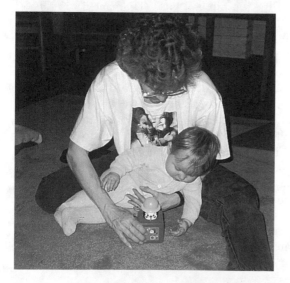

Figure 9–4. Semi-reclined sidelying position with trunk support gives Alex access to this Tomy pop-up clown.

trunk support without interfering with the child's ability to use the arms and hands for reach, grasp, drop, and toy activation (Fig. 9–5). Boppy pillows can be stacked and fastened together with Velcro straps to provide high trunk control for children who will need more than support at the hips and lower trunk. If this low-tech option is insufficient, prop the child into the corner of the couch and offer toys with which to play. Often parents are in the habit of holding a child in sitting position, which can work very well, especially if the parent can be shown where and how to hold the child to provide more or less support for sitting, depending on the child's needs and fatigue level. However, the parent cannot be in front of the child and often cannot see the child's interest in, or reaction to, toys. Offering options that expand sitting choices will give the parents the choice of being behind or in front of the child. When a parent is most comfortable holding the child from behind, the addition of a floor mirror in front of the child will allow parent and child to have visual contact and thereby be able to read each other's visual cues.

For many children, typical high chairs, Sassy Seats, booster seats, and strollers can be adapted with minimal fuss to promote appropriate sitting. Towels can be rolled up and placed on the sides for support; phone books can be covered with contact paper to raise a child to proper height or provide a firmer seat. Dycem may be placed on a seat to prevent sliding forward. Other commercially available seating adaptations may be used to secure a child to a chair (e.g., the Child Safety Sitter Guard, by Rosies Babies) or prevent forward movement (e.g., the Seat Supporter by The Right Start, Fig. 9–6). Numerous assistive devices now more suitable for the young child with significant disabilities are commercially available. See the list of sources in the Appendix.

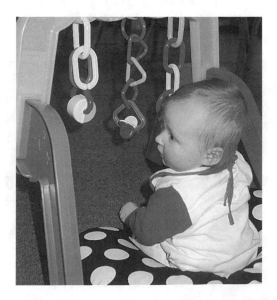

Figure 9–5. The support in sitting provided by the Boppy frees the hands for play.

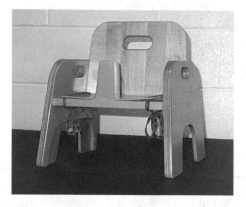

Figure 9–6. The Seat Supporter is shown here attached to a small Rifton chair. The supporter will prevent the pelvis from sliding forward in the seat.

Quadruped

It is unrealistic to expect a child to stay stationary in the quadruped position for any length of time. If the child is typically developing, he or she will move into and out of this position repeatedly, perhaps staying on all fours long enough to rock several times before returning to sitting or prone. Thus, for a child with disabilities, this is considered a transitional position; the adults available should be used as low-tech devices to support the child into and out of this position. Parents able to sit comfortably on the floor can offer a leg to be used much as a therapy roll, with an intriguing toy on one side and the child on the other. Figure 9–7 shows a parent using this position for her 8-month-old child, and the child has come up from all fours to examine the toy (Disney Lights-Go-Round by Disney/Mattel), indicating the transitional nature of this position. Some parents will not find sitting on the floor a comfortable position for play. In this case, rolled up beach towels or therapy rolls can also provide the low-tech option needed to make this work. Guidance and assistance for the child may result in at least brief assumption of the quad-

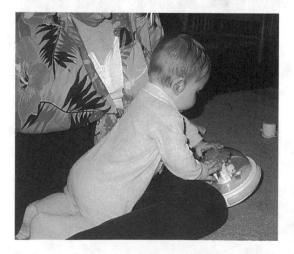

Figure 9–7. Alex adapts the quadruped position for play as he rests his trunk on his mother's leg and plays with the Disney Lights-Go-Round (Disney/Mattel).

ruped position and a return to a more stable position, such as sitting. If the toy requires a hand reach and push to become activated and if the toy has been chosen with the child's interest in mind, the quadruped position may soon give way to a brief three-point position as the child releases one hand to activate the toy.

As noted previously, we encourage the therapist to examine several positioning options for play with the very young child. Typically developing children change positions as often as every second during some aspects of play. This cannot be readily achieved for children with disabilities. Nonetheless, therapists must begin to offer parents and children more than a single "appropriate" position for activities. Using low-technology interventions, positions can more readily be altered as play unfolds if several positioning options have been examined at the outset.

As you begin to develop your own skills for positioning young children for better play, a book you may find helpful is *Positioning for Play*, by R. B. Diamant (1992). This book consists of line drawings for positioning ideas to be used for many activities in many of the positions described previously. In addition, the accompanying text presents simple statements on what skills a specific position will address and what the therapist or parent will need to watch for when using this position. Play ideas are also included. Once you and the parents have determined what positions are optimal for a child, the drawings in this book can be helpful as a reminder to parents. Diamant has used what we have called low-tech positioning in the majority of the book by capitalizing on the parent's body, couch, pillows, boxes, and other readily available items. Rather than reinventing the wheel, therapists may use the pages of this book to show parents positioning options for play. Published by Therapy Skill Builders, the pages of this book may be reproduced for instructional purposes.

TOYS AND SWITCHES

What will make these positions work is not the skill of the parent or even the skill of the therapist, but rather the interest of the child. The child will not be as motivated by the position as by what can be done with and from the position. As noted in Chapter 4, switches and switch-activated toys make the difference for children with significant disabilities between what they can and cannot do and whether or not they can participate in and contribute to an activity. These adaptations, which we include in the category of low-tech, will also have a major impact on the child's motivation to interact with the environment and an impact on how enjoyable an activity is.

Switches and electronic toys are not limited to use by older children. As noted, early learning of concepts such as cause and effect (a skill developed within the 1st year of life in typical children) can be promoted by switch use. Thus, a child who is able to press a switch and watch a battery-operated car move exhibits cause and effect knowledge and demonstrates sensorimotor play level skills. This same child may extend his or her play beyond cause and effect when a tray is placed on the toy car to take a pretend cup of juice to someone in the room. The child is incorporating another individual into the play sequence and engaging in symbolic play. In addition, the child now adds direction following, choice making, sustained motor pressing, and directionality to his or her repertoire of skills. As play complexity is extended, cognitive development is promoted. When such skills are combined with the various positioning options, and possibly with other children, development in many realms can be promoted.

There is some guidance as to appropriate toys and switches for very young children (Williams, Briggs, and Williams, 1979; Newson & Head, 1979). However, therapists will largely need to work with parents and develop their own knowledge base for determining whether or not a child requires a switch with auditory or vibratory feedback, one that is very large, or one that requires very little pressure to activate. The therapist will develop a plan for each child and family that will move the child from activation of the "big red" switch to watch the battery-operated horse move, to pressing the 1-inch square on the Intellikeys communication board to communicate thoughts.

Many resources are available for parents and therapists for making switches and adapting toys. As noted in Chapter 4, it is often time consuming and not always cost-effective to make switches, but it may be a necessity in some cases. Those interested in this skill may want to check such resources as Burkhart (1980, 1982), Wright and Nomura (1985), and Goossens' & Crain (1992). This is not meant to be an exhaustive list, but merely a place to begin.

MOBILITY

Chapter 6 addresses the issue of powered mobility. How does this apply to the very young child? As the author notes, some research evidence supports using powered mobility with the young child, suggesting that very young children can learn to use it and can do so safely. In addition, giving the child mobility has an impact on social-emotional growth and self-image. These reasons alone support the application of this high technology to children at very young ages.

Low-tech mobility options should also be considered. If the child has use of his or her arms for mobility, a scooter board or caster cart may allow greater speed and independence in movement than can be achieved by commando crawling or rolling. Keep in mind Angelo's warning about energy conservation: Just because the child can roll or belly crawl does not mean that this is the most optimal means of mobility throughout the day.

Therapists will need to be open minded and creative when working with parents to establish a means of independent mobility for very young children. It is not so much how the child moves, but that the child has a means of independent mobility that is critical, because this lays essential foundations for development. Environmental exploration is integral in the development of cognition and spatial concepts and for body scheme. Being able to "chase" and "escape" sets the child up for social interactive games with peers and adults. Autonomy has its roots in the 2-year-old behavior of saying "no" and running in the opposite direction. These options can and should be given to the child at a very early age. The choice between high-technology or low-technology mobility will depend on the parental goals, needs, and preferences and the ability of the child.

OTHER TECHNOLOGY DEVICES

Other high-tech devices that may play an appropriate role in promoting development and play in very young children include computers and communication systems (Behrmann, 1984; Butler, 1986; Robinson, 1986; van-Tatenhove, 1987; Swinth, Anson, and Deitz, 1993). Aspects of these devices are reviewed in Chapters 3 and 7. When considering the use of such devices with children younger than 3 years of age, the therapist needs to consider parental goals, preferences, and readiness for complex devices and the skills, goals, and needs of the child. The application of high-tech devices to very young children will be an individual decision.

Thus, our answer to the question posed at the outset of this chapter is most definitely *yes*! The application of technology must be considered for all individuals with disabilities. Assistive technology, and the services needed to support AT are mandated in the public laws that provide for civil rights and a free, appropriate public education for all individuals with disabilities. More than that, technology has the potential to forestall the onset of learned helplessness and to promote play and development in all domains, at all ages.

STUDY QUESTIONS

1. There are many switch-adapted, battery-operated toys available from special catalogues. Make a list of the toys with which you are familiar, and describe the characteristic(s) of the toy that may make it either appealing to the child or potentially aversive. For instance, consider the train that is available that plays loud music. This may be very good for those children in need of loud sound to get their attention, but it may not work well for children who are sensitive to sound.
2. Considering the above characteristics, go shopping at a local toy store and attempt to identify toys that can be adapted to be accessible to a child with a disability that may have similar characteristics.
3. Given your above lists, decide what position(s) the child could use when playing with the toy.

REFERENCES

NICHY News Digest. (1991). The education of children and youth with special needs: What do the laws say? *NICHY News Digest, 1*(1), 1–14.

Athey, I. (1988). The relationship of play to cognitive, language, and moral development. In D. Bergen (Ed.), *Play as a medium for learning and development: A Handbook of theory and practice* (pp. 81–101). Portsmouth, NH: Heinemann.

Behrmann, M. M. (1984). A brighter future for early learning through high tech. *The Pointer, 28*(2), 23–26.

Behrmann, M. M, Jones, J. K., & Wilds, M. (1989). Technology intervention for very young children with disabilities. *Infants and Young Children, 1*(4), 66–77.

Behrmann, M., & Lahm, E. (1984). Babies and robots: Technology to assist learning. *Rehabilitation Literature, 45*(7), 194–201.

Bergen, D. (1991). *Play as the vehicle for early intervention with at-risk infants and toddlers.* Paper presented at the annual meeting of the American Educational Research Association, Chicago, IL.

Bradley, M. P. (1994). Computers for the very young: From the ridiculous to the sublime. *Closing the Gap, 13*(2), 1–5.

Bradley, R. H. (1985). Social-cognitive development and toys. *Topics in Early Childhood Special Education, 5*(3), 11–30.

Brinker, R. P., & Lewis, M. (1982). Making the world work with microcomputers: A learning prosthesis for handicapped infants. *Exceptional Children, 49*(2), 163–170.

Burkhart, L. (1980). *Homemade battery-powered toys and educational devices for severely handicapped children.* Eldersburg, MD: Author.

Burkhart, L. (1982). *More homemade battery devices for severely handicapped children with suggestions,* Eldersburg, MD: Author.

Butler, C. (1986). Effects of powered mobility on self-initiated behaviors of very young children with locomotor disability. *Developmental Medicine & Child Neurology, 28,* 325–332.

Butler, C. (1988), High tech toys: Technology for mobility, manipulation, communication, and learning in early childhood. *Infants and Young Children: An Interdisciplinary Journal for Special Care Practices, 1*(2), 66–73.

Curry, N., & Bergen, D. (1988), The relationship of play to emotional, social, and gender/sex role development. In D. Bergen (Ed.), *Play as a medium for learning and development: A handbook of theory and practice* (pp. 107–131). Portsmouth, NH: Heinemann.

Diamant, R. B. (1992). *Positioning for Play.* Tuscon: Therapy Skill Builders.

Douglas, J., Reeson, B., & Ryan, M. (1988). Computer microtechnology for a severely disabled preschool child. *Child: Care, Health, and Development, 14*(2), 93–104.

Florey, L. (1971). An approach to play and play development. *The American Journal of Occupational Therapy, 15*(6), 275–280.

Gallagher, J. J., Trohanis, P. L., & Clifford, R. M. (1989). *Policy Implementation and PL 99-457.* Baltimore: Paul H. Brooks Publishing.

Goosens', C, & Crain, S. S. (1992). *Utilizing switch interfaces with children who are severely physically challenged.* Austin, TX: ProEd.

Hanson, M. J., & Hanline, M. F. (1985). An analysis of response-contingent learning experiences for young children. *The Journal of the Association for Persons with Severe Handicaps, 10*(1), 31–40.

Jennings, K. D., Connors, R. E., Stegman, C. E., Sankaranarayan, P., & Medolsohn (1985). Mastery motivation in young preschoolers. *Journal of the Division of Early Childhood, 9*(2), 162–169.

Kaplan, J., & Kopp, C. (1983). The effect of developmental delay on sustained attention in young children. *Child Development, 54,* 1143–1155.

Kaplan-Sanoff, M., Brewster, A., Stillwell, J., & Bergen, D. (1988). The relationship of play to physical/motor development and to children with special needs. In D. Bergen (Ed.), *Play as a medium for learning and development: A handbook of theory and practice.* (pp. 137–161). Portsmouth, NH: Heinemann.

Langley, M. B. (1990). A developmental approach to the use of toys for facilitation of environmental control. *Physical & Occupational Therapy in Pediatrics, 10*(2), 69–91.

Li, A. K. F. (1981). Play and the mentally retarded. *Mental Retardation, 19,* 121–126.

Newson, E., & Head, J. (1979). Play and playthings for the handicapped child. In J. Newson & E. Newson (Eds.). *Toys and Playthings in Development and Remediation* (pp. 140–214). London: Dearge Allen & Unwin.

Robinson, L. M. (1986). Designing computer intervention for very young handicapped children. *Journal of the Division for Early Childhood, 10*(3), 209–215.

Swinth, Y., Anson, D., & Deitz, J. (1993). Single-switch computer access for infants and toddlers. *The American Journal of Occupational Therapy, 47*(11), 1031–1038.

vanTatenhove, G. (1987). Teaching power through augmentative communication: Guidelines for early intervention. *Journal of Childhood Communication Disorders, 10*(2), 185–199.

Wachs, T. D., & Gruen, G. (1982). *Early experience and human development.* New York: Plenum Press.

Warren, S. F., & Horn, E. M. (1987). Microcomputer applications in early childhood special education: Problems and possibilities. *Topics in Early Childhood Special Education, 7*(2), 72–84.

Wilds, M. L. (1989). Effective use of technology with young children. *NICHCY News Digest, 13,* 6–7.

Williams, B., Briggs, N., & Williams, R. (1979). Selecting, adapting, and understanding toys and reaction. In P. Wehman (Ed.), *Recreation programming for developmentally disabled persons* (pp. 15–36). Baltimore: University Park Press.

Williams, S. E., & Matesi, D. V. (1988). Therapeutic intervention with an adapted toy. *The American Journal of Occupational Therapy, 42*(10), 673–676.

Wright, C., & Nomura, M. (1985). *From Toys to Computers.* San Jose, CA: Author.

Selected Sources for Assistive Devices for the Very Young Child

Childcraft
PO Box 3081
Edison, NJ 08818
1-800-631-5652

Chime Time
2440-C Pleasantdale Road
Atlanta, GA 30340-1562
1-800-477-5075

Computability Corp.
40000 Grand River, Suite #109
Novi, MN 48050
(313) 477-6720

Community Playthings
Box 901
Rifton, NY 12471-0901
1-800-777-4244

Constructive Playthings
1227 East 119th Street
Grandview, MO 64030-1117
1-800-448-4115

Crestwood Co.
6625 North Sidney Place
Milwaukee, WI 53209
(414) 352-5678

Funtastic Therapy
RD #4 Box 14
Cranberry, NJ 08512
1-800-531-3176

Jesana, Ltd.,
PO Box 17
Irvington, NY 10533
1-800-443-4728

Kapable Kids
PO Box 250
Bohemia, NY 11716
1-800-356-1564

Lakeshore Learning
2695 East Dominque Street
Carson, CA 90749
1-800-421-5354

One Step Ahead
PO Box 517
Lake Bluff, IL 60044
1-800-274-8440

Right Start Catalog
Right Start Plaza
5334 Sterling Center Drive
Westlake Village, CA 91361-4627
1-800-548-8531

Sammons Pediatric Catalog
145 Tower Drive
Burr Ridge, IL 60521
1-800-323-5547

Southpaw Enterprise
109 Webb Street
Dayton, OH 45403-1144
1-800-228-1698

Sportime Abilitations
One Sportime Way
Atlanta, GA 30340
1-800-845-1535

Toys to Grow On
PO Box 17
Long Beach, CA 90801
1-800-542-8338

Toys for Special Children
385 Warburton Avenue
Hasting-on-Hudson, NY 10706
914-478-0960

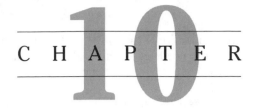

CHAPTER 10

FUNDING

Lewis Golinker, Esquire, and Susan G. Mistrett, MS, Ed

Assistive Technology Guide

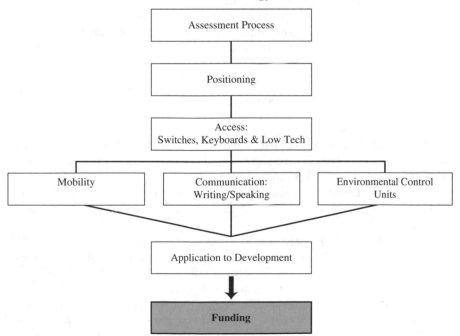

211

A core function of occupational therapists (OTs) and physical therapists (PTs) is to identify a client's need for assistive devices. Like all other forms of OT and PT services, assistive devices enhance client functioning, which in turn improves quality of life.

Obtaining funding for assistive devices, or assistive technology (AT) devices as they now are called by some funding programs, is also an inherent part of the OT's and PT's role. The recommended equipment will be as much for the client's benefit as any other OT or PT service. Obtaining funding for the equipment is therefore critical, even though the flow of dollars may pass from the funding program to an equipment vendor, rather than directly to or through the therapist. In addition, the therapist must apply the same skills when seeking funding for equipment as for the therapist's own services: application of a high degree of a professional skill to conduct the assessment and make the recommendation; preparation of accurate, complete, and program-responsive documentation; and in many cases, advocacy on behalf of the recommendation, until a favorable response is obtained.

The bottom line is that without funding, nothing happens. Unless funding is provided to transform on-paper recommendations into tangible services and devices, the most expert therapy evaluation and the most comprehensive and articulate treatment and services plans will be meaningless. Without funding, a treatment plan will not be implemented. Therapy services and assistive devices will not be provided. The goals for functional improvement stated in the treatment plan will remain just that—goals.

This chapter provides a general introduction to three benefits and services programs that will provide funding for assistive devices recommended by OTs and PTs: Medicaid, private health insurance, and public education. It outlines the purpose for each program and how funding justifications can be structured. This chapter also identifies other resources to assist therapists with funding challenges.

MEDICAID

Medicaid is also known as "medical assistance" or "Title XIX." Medicaid was created in 1965 to enable people who are poor and people with disabilities to access health care services they otherwise would not be able to afford. It is a publicly funded program, with the costs split between the federal and state governments. Medicaid provides reimbursement for the cost of health care services provided to more than 35 million people, half of whom are children.

Medicaid is administered as 56 separate programs (including the 50 states, the District of Columbia, and five U.S. territories). Federal mandates impose a core of eligibility and benefits requirements, which result in common features for all Medicaid programs throughout the country. In addition, the individual states have discretion to shape their programs to fit their individual circumstances (i.e., by covering additional low-income individuals and providing additional medical services). As a result, there will be some variation from state to state regarding populations served and benefits provided by their Medicaid programs.

Understanding and Properly Applying Medicaid Vocabulary Is Essential

Therapists must become familiar with the key Medicaid terms used in this chapter. While Medicaid has the potential to be a major source of funding for assistive devices, the failure to adopt standard Medicaid vocabulary will almost certainly increase the risk of unnecessary funding delays or denials.

Assistive Technology Is Not Within the Medicaid Vocabulary

The first and perhaps most important lesson regarding Medicaid vocabulary is that the phrase "assistive technology device" is **not** used by Medicaid except in one or two limited circumstances and should not be used in funding justifications or other documentation submitted to Medicaid. Assistive Technology devices are identified by name as available services within the Medicaid provisions for "home and community based waivers," authorized by Section 1915 C of the Social Security Act, 42 USC § 1396n(g), and the Medicaid provisions for "community supported living arrangements" (CSLA) 42 USC § 1396d(a) (23). At present, the CSLA program is in effect only in California, Colorado, Florida, Illinois, Maryland, Michigan, Rhode Island, and Wisconsin. All Medicaid documentation should identify the specific device being requested by name, and the only descriptive terms used should match a word or phrase from the definition of one of the Medicaid services from which the device or equipment is being sought.

Funding Barriers

In some Medicaid programs and for some assistive devices, funding will be based on clear criteria. For a substantial percentage of Medicaid beneficiaries, however, obtaining assistive devices will be more difficult. Seven common funding barriers follow:

1. The lack of definitions for essential terms, such as durable medical equipment, and prosthetic devices
2. The lack of any criteria related to the standard of "medical need"
3. The lack of any reference list of covered equipment
4. The existence of a list of covered or noncovered items that is significantly out of date or incomplete
5. The existence of a list of covered and noncovered items that includes similar equipment on both lists
6. A lack of knowledge, skill, and discretion among Medicaid decision makers
7. Application errors of whatever definitions and standards that exist

These barriers are as unnecessary as they are common. They are a fact of life when working with the Medicaid program. As a result, therapists must be prepared to take the steps that will minimize the occurrence of these barriers, and be prepared to take the additional steps that may be necessary to break through them.

In general, the operating presumption for OTs and PTs when dealing with Medicaid programs is that assistive devices determined to be necessary to aid the functional independence of Medicaid beneficiaries *are* covered and *will* be funded. Therapists should maintain the expectation that their clients will be granted the assistive device(s) they require.

Key Questions

Three key questions should be addressed by a therapist requesting Medicaid funding. They are as follows:

Does the Menu of Services Offered by That State's Medical Program Include Services That "Cover" Assistive Devices?

Medicaid coverage of specific services may be "mandatory" or "optional." Mandatory Medicaid services *must* be provided by all states as part of their participation in the Medicaid program. The mandatory Medicaid services follow:

- Inpatient and outpatient hospital care
- Physicians' services
- Laboratory and x-ray services
- Nurse-midwife services
- Rural health clinic services
- Early periodic screening, diagnosis and treatment for people younger than 21 years of age
- Home health care services to people older than 21 years of age, including medical supplies and equipment
- Services to pregnant women
- Family planning services and supplies to individuals of childbearing age
- Skilled nursing facility services for people older than 21 years of age (42 USC § 1396a; 1396d[a])

Optional services, as their name implies, *may* be selected by each state Medicaid program at their discretion and made available to their Medicaid beneficiaries. States are able to select optional services from a list included in the federal Medicaid Act. If selected, the states receive the same level of federal assistance as for their mandatory Medicaid services (i.e., between 50% and 80% of the cost of the service). States also have substantial flexibility in their decision to add or delete optional services from their programs. The optional services available to states include:

- Podiatrist, optometrist, chiropractor, or other practitioners services
- Private duty nursing
- Clinic services
- Dental services
- Occupational, physical, speech, hearing, and language therapy and other rehabilitative services
- Prescribed drugs
- Christian Science schools
- Nursing facilities for people younger than 21 years of age
- Emergency hospital services
- Personal care services
- Hospice care
- Case management services
- Eyeglasses
- Diagnostic and screening services
- Preventive services
- Transportation services
- Services for people 65 years or older in mental institutions
- Intermediate care facility services
- Inpatient psychiatric services for people younger than 22 years of age (42 USC § 1396d[a])

Note that "assistive devices" is not identified as a separate Medicaid service and it is not found on either of these services lists. Yet assistive devices *are* within the scope of the Medicaid program in every state.

Absent an express reference, the starting point to identify the basis for Medicaid assistive device funding must be the federal Medicaid definitions of these Medicaid services. The federal definitions explain the intent and scope of each Medicaid service. In addition, the federal definitions are applicable to all Medicaid programs, and all services, whether mandatory or optional; as a condition of participation, states must comply with the definitions and requirements of the federal Medicaid law and rules.

Because the basis for coverage of assistive devices will be the *federal* Medicaid regulations, which are not subject to state control, therapists should not start their inquiry about Medicaid with a phone call to the state Medicaid program or even with a search of a state Medicaid provider manual. These state sources may not accurately or reliably describe the required scope of Medicaid assistive device coverage.

A review of the federal Medicaid regulations identifies eight services among the list of mandatory and optional services that are the primary sources for funding of assistive devices. These services follow:

- Early and periodic screening, diagnostic and treatment services
- Home health care services
- Prosthetic devices
- Occupational therapy services
- Physical therapy services
- Rehabilitative services
- Skilled nursing facility
- Services and Intermediate Care Facility Services for Persons with Mental Retardation, Developmental Disabilities, and related conditions (ICF/MR-DD)

Through one or more of these Medicaid services, OTs and PTs have been able to recommend and obtain Medicaid funding for devices related to the following:

- Improved seating and positioning
- Mobility
- Client safety and hygiene
- Lifts
- Environmental control units
- Splints, braces, prosthetic devices, and orthotic devices
- Augmentative communication devices

The second and third questions faced by occupational and physical therapists seeking Medicaid funding for assistive devices concern the procedural and substantive standards and limitations, if any, that affect device access and funding.

What Procedural Requirements or Limitations Apply to These Medicaid Services?

Prior Approval

Access to OT and PT services and almost all devices under any of the service categories listed previously will most likely be governed by a "prior approval" or "prior authorization" process. This procedure requires a recipient to request that Medicaid approve the service or device for funding in advance of its being provided. The request explains why the therapy service or device is "medically necessary."

In many states, prior approval is not required for *all* OT and PT services. Instead, some amount of therapy (i.e., some number of occupational and physical therapy sessions) are permitted to be provided based solely on a doctor's prescription. Any therapy greater than that threshold will be subject to a prior approval review. Other states require prior approval for all therapy services. Almost all states require prior approval for all but the most common Medicaid-funded devices and equipment.

Submission of prior approval requests is the responsibility of the service provider, who may be the therapist. Although the prior approval documents are not complicated, they must be prepared with great care.

Funding Justifications

All Medicaid services for all beneficiaries (children and adults) must be "medically necessary." Medical need is a term of art in the Medicaid program, but no federal Medicaid regulation defines it. Instead, definitions of medical need are left to the states, but not all states have clearly written definitions.

As a general rule, the medical need for an assistive device will be based on five common factors. To establish medical need, a funding justification for a device should address *all* of the following points:

1. Describe the recipient's diagnosis or condition that can be connected specifically to the functional impairment that will be addressed by the device. For augmentative or alternative communication (AAC) devices, specific speech-language diagnoses must be used (e.g., dysarthria, apraxia, aphasia, rather than "cerebral palsy" or "stroke"). For seating, positioning, and mobility devices, comparable specific diagnoses should be used, rather than global descriptive terms, such as spastic quadriplegia. Chandler (1992) suggests that OTs make it clear that they are treating the functional disability, which occurs secondary to the primary diagnosis. For example, although OTs treat many children with cerebral palsy, they do not treat the cerebral palsy. Instead, they address the functional disabilities that result from the primary diagnosis of cerebral palsy.

2. Describe the specific adverse functional effects (functional limitations) caused by the diagnosis or condition that will be addressed by the device. Describe thoroughly how the recipient is unable to perform certain tasks as a direct result of the diagnosis or condition.

3. A. Identify and describe the device in specific terms and with all its necessary features, accessories, or customization.
   B. Describe the device as a form of treatment for the condition or diagnosis.
   C. Describe the evaluation of need and the recommendation of this device as treatment as being within the recognized scope of practice of occupational or physical therapists.

4. Describe specifically the effect of the device or service—that it will alleviate or ameliorate (lessen the severity of) or eliminate the adverse functional limitations or the disabling effects (described in item 2) caused by the diagnosis or condition. Do not use general, subjective phrases, such as "improve independence" or "improve quality of life." Use only terminology related to functional improvements to overcome physiologic limitations.

5. Explain and provide an analysis of the process by which you conclude that the device being recommended is the least costly alternative form of treatment that will provide the effects described in item 4.

The American Occupational Therapy Association (AOTA) approved a position paper on *Occupational Therapy and Assistive Technology* (AOTA, 1991). This position paper should be attached, excerpted, or referenced in all funding justifications for assistive devices. It is essential that the therapist not use the term "assistive technology" to describe the device being requested from Medicaid. Medicaid does not use that phrase in its vocabulary and will almost certainly reject requests that describe a device using it.

Therapist Experience

Funding justifications must address with care the specific expertise of the therapist. This is among the most important of all the data supplied to Medicaid in support of a funding request, yet it is frequently the data to which the least attention is paid. Too often, therapists mistakenly believe their letterhead and the initials after their name are sufficient to establish their expertise. It is absolutely essential that Medicaid appellate decision makers are given as much information as possible to show that the professionals supporting the funding request are, without question, more skilled and more expert than the Medicaid staff in their knowledge of the following:

1. The person with a disability
2. The nature, severity, treatment options, and predictable treatment outcomes for the disability at the level of severity experienced by the person
3. The ability of therapy treatment in general and of the specific assistive device requested to treat the disability
4. The ability of other, similar, and potentially less costly devices or other forms of treatment than the one selected to treat the disability

Reliability and credibility of the therapist are essential factors in Medicaid services advocacy. Establishing the therapist's credibility and reliability should focus on the therapist's postschool experience, not his or her college and graduate degrees. Consider the following six points when preparing a funding justification:

1. General professional experience: Describe the therapist's general experience in the field. This will include the number of years of service and an estimate of the number of people evaluated or otherwise served.
2. Experience related to assistive devices: Explain why the therapist believes he or she is qualified to make the assistive device recommendation. Points to consider include the following:

   ■ Classroom learning about technology assessment and selection
   ■ Clinical internships

- Professional education journals related to technology assessment and recommendation that have been reviewed; technology-related professional education programs attended
- Professional journal contributions related to technology
- Continuing education program presentations related to technology
- Number of clients evaluated in regard to technology
- Number of devices, systems, and services recommended
- History of public or third-party funding (Therapists whose opinions are respected by other public or third-party funding programs should also have their opinions respected by Medicaid.)
- Basis for familiarity with the range of technology devices and services that may be available

3. Description of the evaluation process: Describe what was done to reach the recommendation. Consider the following:

- Who referred the client? (If the therapist is recognized by his or her peers as having unique, technology-related skills or experience, this should be reported.)
- What information was reviewed about the client prior to the evaluation? What records were reviewed; who was interviewed (clinical records; medical records; school records; parent, caregiver, client interview)? Are the data reviewed about this client similar to those available for others? (It is better that the therapist's data-gathering process and assessment of data follow a standard practice.)
- Where did the evaluation occur? (A clinic- or rehabilitation center–based assessment will be more professionally credible than a home evaluation, particularly to establish that alternative devices were considered.)
- How long did the evaluation take, and was the time devoted to the evaluation comparable to that given to others?
- Did the evaluation follow a standardized protocol? Was this inquiry procedure developed by a professional organization (e.g., AOTA) has the professional personally created or adapted it from a professional protocol; does the professional use this technique all the time; how many evaluations have been done using this inquiry technique?
- What was done? (Describe briefly.)
- Has this evaluation process led to recommendations for devices that were funded by Medicaid in the past or by other public or third-party funding sources? If Medicaid or other payers have approved the same device in the past, this is a very important point to add.

4. Evaluation results: Describe the client's current mental and physical condition and his or her lifestyle. This discussion must be detailed: this portion of the report identifies the person's *medical need*.
5. The selection process: Medicaid expects therapists to have considered a range of devices, including no device, as alternative means to ad-

dress the person's functional limitations. Consider the following points to describe the process of selecting the assistive devices being recommended:

■ What devices and services were considered as alternatives, and why were the alternatives rejected?
■ Was there a trial-use period? If so, was the trial a success?

When this information is provided, Medicaid decision makers at all levels will have a sufficient basis to conclude that the therapist's opinion regarding the appropriateness of the assistive device is reliable and that the device should be approved.

Medicaid makes it mandatory that therapists consider the least costly alternative treatment service or device capable of achieving a particular outcome. As applied in the Medicaid program, an alternative is a service, device, or strategy that will yield the same, or a substantially similar, degree of functional improvement as some other service, device, or strategy. The key point in the comparison is the level of functional improvement that can be achieved.

There is no objective way to compare assistive devices regarding features or cost. When one device has a feature and another does not, it is important to explain how the features of the recommended device are, or will be, meaningful to the user. However, it is not necessary that every feature have current value. Some may come into use in the future. For those, the funding justification must explain how that "future" is reasonably foreseeable in the user's and device's useful life.

6. The Recommendation: The features of the assistive device being recommended must be described. In particular, the therapist must explain clearly that the client needs and will use all the components of the device or system. The device or system must be shown to match the person's abilities, limitations, and needs.

Ultimately, the narrative report touching on all these subjects will be a few pages long and may take a few hours to prepare. However, the effort will be well worth it, because funding will not be approved without it.

Do Any Restrictions on Medicaid's Ability to Impose Amount, Duration, and Scope Limitations Apply?

Three general rules limit the freedom of state Medicaid programs from severely restricting access to devices within the covered services we have been discussing. These limitations arise from the Medicaid program and the Americans with Disabilities Act.

The first program limitation is that Medicaid is required to provide all services in "sufficient amount, duration, and scope to reasonably achieve their purposes" (42 CFR § 440.238[b]). Second, Medicaid is permitted to establish rules that limit services based on the degree of medical need (42 CFR § 440.230[d]). And third, Medicaid programs are forbidden from restricting specific forms of treatment within covered services based on diagnosis, type of illness, or condition (42 CFR § 440.230[c]).

These rules restrict Medicaid's freedom to make any covered service meaningless (i.e., of no benefit) to a recipient (Pinnecke v. Preisser 623 F.2d 546 8th Cir., 1980). As applied to assistive devices and other equipment, Medicaid is not permitted to provide prosthetic devices that will address some nonfunctioning or malfunctioning body parts but not others. For example, for a person needing an AAC device, Medicaid is not permitted to limit the scope of prosthetic devices to those capable of meeting the needs of people with missing, nonfunctioning, or malfunctioning upper and lower limbs but not nonfunctioning or malfunctioning oral–motor mechanisms. Medicaid is not permitted to provide coverage for an artificial larynx, which is one form of AAC device, and not also provide funding for other AAC devices, such as the Liberator and DynaVox. In regard to mobility, these rules prohibit Medicaid from approving payment for manual wheelchairs and at the same time denying payment for powered wheelchairs.

For individuals older than 21 years of age, Medicaid does have the flexibility to set "useful life" rules, which will be stated as an interval that must pass before a new device of the same type can be requested. But these rules must be tied to some reasonable statement of the anticipated useful life of an item of equipment; and they must be flexible enough to permit replacement of a device when required due to a change in the person's condition.

When a person's condition and needs change or the device breaks and is not capable of being repaired, the person is left in the position of having no device currently able to meet his or her needs. In these circumstances, a repair should occur, or a new device should be provided. Medicaid may inquire closely about how and why the person's needs have changed so sufficiently to render the existing device unusable or how and why the device was broken, but in the final analysis, the device should be repaired or replaced. The therapist may need to develop the argument in support of this replacement.

PRIVATE HEALTH INSURANCE

The extraordinary costs associated with health care make private health care a highly prized benefit in contemporary American society. For all Americans, having a source of health care payment, such as insurance or a health benefits plan, provides a measure of financial security, which may spell the difference between family financial stability and insolvency.

For people with disabilities and their family members, the value of this benefit is unique. Health insurance or benefits plan coverage can be the difference between treatment that supports independent functioning and care at home and dependency and institutionalization. These issues are not shared by the public; they are unique to the life experiences of people with disabilities and their families.

Assistive devices are another unique need of people with disabilities, and they are a benefit of health care payment sources that is meaningful only to them. Health insurance and benefits plans have been, and should continue to be, a major supplier of assistive devices in the United States. These sources have provided coverage for augmentative communication devices, bath safety equipment (e.g., shower and bath chairs and lifts), specialized beds (e.g., hospital beds and special mattresses), environmental control devices, hearing aids, individual lifts, mobility devices (including canes, walkers, manual wheelchairs and powered vehicles, such as three-wheeled scooters), and seating and positioning devices (e.g., custom seating systems, standing frames, seat-lift chairs). This equipment represents a sample, not an encyclopedic list of the types of devices that have been provided through private health care coverage.

Unfortunately, there is no mandate for universal coverage either for people or for services. As to services, there is no common benefits list applicable to all insurance policies or health benefits plans. As a result, each person must review the documents related to his or her own health care coverage to determine its scope.

What Is Covered by a Health Care Policy or Benefits Plan

The procedures for interpreting insurance and health plan documents are generally the same as those applied to Medicaid. As with Medicaid, the starting point for reviewing a health insurance policy, benefits booklet, or health benefits plan description is to have a set of expectations about the outcome of the funding process. It is reasonable to expect that a health insurance policy or benefits plan *should* cover AT devices that people with disabilities or their family members require. When such devices or services are denied, the most simple and straightforward response is to ask, "Why?"

This is the most powerful of all possible responses. Insurers and plan administrators may not expect questions about their decisions and may resist providing responses, but the expectation of "yes" should push you to be insistent. If the request for a device is denied and reasons such as "not medically necessary," "not medical equipment," or "requested item is a convenience item" are supplied, the therapist should obtain further information. Inquire as to where in the policy or benefits plan durable or prosthetic medical equipment devices are found; find out how and where they are defined. Also ask for examples of devices that fit those terms and how those devices satisfy the criteria.

It then is the therapist's responsibility to craft a response. In all circumstances, the response must show that the device being sought satisfies any applicable criteria. But the therapist must be prepared for the possibility that the devices being requested are not specifically listed in any policy or plan documents, or that the service where the device will be found (e.g., DME or prosthetic devices) is not defined. Or, the policy or plan may define the service by reference to general criteria, as does Medicaid, but there is no explanation why the device being requested fails to satisfy those criteria. Yet another variation is that examples of covered equipment are provided, but not the specific device being requested. Regardless of which of these (or other) circumstances are presented, the therapist must explain how these criteria are met. Ultimately, the therapist's efforts to provide ongoing responses and to continue to push the insurer or plan administrator to explain "why not" have a good chance of being rewarded with success. Perseverence, however frustrating, pays off.

As noted previously, therapists seeking to provide assistive devices to people with disabilities must answer the same questions regarding coverage and access that arise with Medicaid. Therapists should refer to that section of this chapter to answer the following key issues:

- Whether the scope of benefits includes OT and PT services, assistive devices, durable medical equipment or orthotics, and prosthetic devices
- Whether there are specific definitions for these services or for general services for access criteria, such as "medical need"
- Whether there are specific limitations on amount, duration, and scope of services or devices
- What the procedure used and documentation required are to access covered services

Follow All Stated Procedures

In general, access to assistive devices will require a physician's prescription, supported by a funding justification prepared by an OT or PT. The justification must explain how the device is a covered service, and it must describe the medical need for the device, just as is required by Medicaid.

If the insurer or plan administrator rejects the request for funding, there is likely to be a procedure for appeal. In all circumstances, therapists are encouraged to seek the assistance of advocacy resources.

Appeals often are written statements explaining why the adverse funding decision was improper and adding any further information that may have been omitted in the initial application. The appeal also should make clear the applicant's belief that the policy or plan does cover the requested device and that the rejection was inconsistent with the policy or plan. At this point, funding approvals by sources such as Medicaid and other policies or plans are important facts to add to initial funding justifications and appeals.

In addition, four other points should be addressed:

- Have all the documentation requirements stated in the policy or plan been followed? Have all of the necessary forms, justifications, and so forth been submitted? If not, these documents must be supplied.
- The appeal letter should make specific reference to the covered service(s) that will support funding (therapy, durable medical equipment, prosthetics), and the insurer or plan administrator should be asked specifically to explain why coverage is not available under any and all of these services.
- Some insurance companies limit coverage of durable medical equipment to U.S. Food and Drug Administration (FDA)–approved devices. Many seating, positioning, and mobility devices have received FDA approval. The therapist can get this information from a device manufacturer or vendor. The appeal letter should make specific reference to the fact that the device being requested is a medical device approved by the FDA.
- Insurance companies often use Medicare as a comparable funding source (i.e., if Medicare will cover the item, then the insurer will too). Therapists should seek information about past Medicare practice from the equipment vendor and from the advocacy resources listed at the end of this chapter. In any case in which a funding source states an assistive device is not covered because Medicare will not cover it, an independent inquiry about Medicare's payment practices should be undertaken.

As with Medicaid, in many cases, appeals lead to the reversal of adverse funding decisions.

Issues Related to Services and Devices Available From Other Funding Sources at No Charge

Insurance policies and benefits plans, like all other funding sources, may try to position themselves as the payer of last resort. These may be written as coverage limitations stating the following:

- Services that can be obtained without charge from any other funding source are not covered.
- For people between the ages of 3 and 21 years of age, a specific list of services is not covered if they are required to be provided between the hours of 8 AM and 3 PM.

The first limitation is designed to force people to use government benefits before seeking payment from their insurance policy. The second is specifically designed to force children to use the special education program as the primary payer for required health services. The list of excluded services will parallel the list of related services in the Individuals with Disabilities Education Act (IDEA).

Therapists should be alert to these insurance policy or benefits plan statements. The federal Medicaid Act forbids attempts by these sources to require prior application to Medicaid; it states that all third-party funding sources, including insurance policies and benefits plans, must be used to their maximum before Medicaid can be tapped. No insurance policy can exempt itself from that federal law. Although self-insuring employers are exempt from *state* regulation of health benefits, they are not exempt from *federal* laws and rules.

The second limitation presents a different set of concerns. First, limitations of this type are legal. They were unsuccessfully challenged by school districts as being against public policy. The schools argued that the IDEA expressly states that schools may look to insurance as a source of funding for a child's free and appropriate public education (FAPE); if insurers simply can write themselves out of any responsibility, then the intent of these IDEA cost-sharing provisions would be defeated. However, the courts agreed with the insurers. Neither the IDEA nor any other law directs them to include certain services in their policies; thus, they can write their policies any way they want without regard to their fiscal impact on the schools.

Limitations of this type assume that schools will provide therapy and assistive devices whenever they are needed because they are within the IDEA's scope. Unfortunately, that does not always occur. When schools refuse to provide services or devices, the therapist must go back to the insurer or plan administrator to seek payment for the needed services and devices.

PUBLIC EDUCATION

The third source of funding to consider is within the public education system. To understand funding for AT within this system, one must first understand the public education laws that define and describe AT devices and services.

Public Education Laws Affecting Assistive Technology Funding

Several federal laws impact the educational programs and services that children with disabilities receive. Specifically, these laws address their education and civil rights by guaranteeing that all students receive a FAPE. These laws can be described as impacting the services that students with disabilities receive (including those related to AT), their educational setting, or both.

The Individuals with Disabilities Education Act (P.L. 101-476), formerly known as the Education for All Handicapped Children Act (EHA, P.L. 94-142), and its amendments identify the special education and related services mandated for students with disabilities to receive their FAPE. In addition, section 504 of the Rehabilitation Act of 1973 protects the rights of students with disabilities not requiring special education services to have full access to all programs and activities offered by the school. Both laws support the right of students with disabilities to use AT devices and services to meet their educational needs.

This legislation continues to mandate FAPE for all students with disabilities and ensures their rights and those of their parents or guardians. Appropriate education is the provision of regular and special education and related services designed to meet the individual educational needs of students; this encourages the child to be educated with nondisabled children. These services must be free and provided by the school district at no cost to the parents. Due process procedures are guaranteed so that parents or guardians can review and participate in decisions made for their child.

To ensure that each program is determined on a case-by-case basis to meet the unique needs of each student, an individualized education program (IEP) is developed for each child by a multidisciplinary team. It is based on a full assessment and addresses the child's current level of ability, stating the special education and related services he or she will receive.

Since 1974, the EHA has guaranteed educational opportunities for children with disabilities, ages 5 to 21 years. In 1986, an amendment to the EHA, required that states extend the rights to FAPE to children from 3 to 5 years old by providing special education and related services. It also established a new, voluntary state program for providing early intervention services for infants and toddlers with disabilities from birth to 2 years of age. This amendment, P.L. 99-457, significantly expanded the rights and entitlements of young children with disabilities. For infants and toddlers with disabilities, an individual family service plan (IFSP) is developed to state the type of services each child and family will receive.

In 1990, amendments were again added to the EHA. The amendment replaced the phrase "handicapped child" with "child with a disability," and changed the name of the law to the Individuals with Disabilities Education Act (P.L. 101-476). Substantively, the IDEA strengthened children's rights to access assistive devices that always were part of the concept of "free appropriate public education" under P.L. 94-142, but never before had been identified specifically in either the law or program rules.

The IDEA accomplishes this by expressly incorporating the terms "assistive technology device" and "assistive technology service," and provides the same definitions as were stated in an earlier federal law known as the Tech Act, or more formally, the Technology Related Assistance for Individuals with Disabilities Act of 1988 (P.L. 100-407). These definitions are as follows:

> *Assistive technology device:* Any item, piece of equipment, or product system, whether acquired commercially off the shelf, modified, or customized, that is used to increase, maintain, or improve functional capabilities of individuals with disabilities

> *Assistive technology service:* Any service that directly assists an individual with a disability in the selection, acquisition, or use of an AT device

Two years later, regulations implementing the IDEA were promulgated which expressly state AT devices and services may be "special education," "related services," or "supplemental aids or services" that comprise the individualized education program for a child with a disability. (34 CFR § 300.308.)

Assistive technology services include the following:

- Evaluation of technology needs in the individual's customary environment
- Acquisition of AT devices
- Selecting, adapting, repairing, or replacing AT devices
- Coordinating and using AT with other therapies, interventions, or services
- Training for AT for an individual or family
- Training for professionals involved with the child's program

The two-pronged definition is important because it places equal value on AT services and equipment. By focusing on just the device, one assumes that this alone will make a difference in a child's ability to be more independent. However, this combination of a carefully selected device and its use by a child with support of parents and professionals in appropriate situations creates opportunities for a child's increased participation and independence.

In the IDEA, children with disabilities, from birth through 21 years of age, must be considered for AT use when it is needed to receive FAPE. AT devices and services must be available to a child with a disability when required as part of the child's special education services, related services, or supplementary aids and services, and a statement of their use must be included on the IEP or IFSP.

Provisions Within the Laws That Support Assistive Technology

Six IDEA provisions are viewed as supporting AT funding: free education, special education, related services, least restrictive environment, procedural safeguards, and staff development (RESNA, 1992). In compliance with these and other services provided through special education legislation, AT devices and services must be considered for all children and be identified by a multidisciplinary team. The use of such devices must be determined within the natural environment, the one in which the device will be used. Statement of their use must be specifically worded on the IEP, and such devices and services must be provided at no cost to the family.

Several policy letters from the Office of Special Education and Rehabilitative Services (OSERS) have clarified the rights of a child with a disability to AT devices and services under IDEA. These clarifications have strengthened the relationship between AT and existing educational provisions. They include the following:

OSERS, 1990 (Goodman letter)

- Student need for AT must be determined on a case-by-case basis.

- The IEP must include a specific statement of AT devices and services, including the nature and the amount of such services.
- The school district is responsible for providing AT at no cost to the parents.

OSERS, 1991

- If the IEP team determines that a particular AT item is required for home use for a child to be provided FAPE, the technology must be provided to implement the IEP.
- The school board may not change the statement of special education and related services contained in the IEP.

OSERS, 1993 (Seiler letter)

- A hearing aid is considered an AT device. When a child with a disability requires a hearing aid to receive FAPE and the child's IEP specifies that the child needs a hearing aid, it must be provided by the school district.

OSERS, 1993 (Moore letter)

- School district funds can be used to purchase a computer for a student with disabilities attending a parochial school if the computer is provided to assist the child to receive FAPE, not for religious instruction.

OSERS, 1994

- If a parent provides an AT device for the IEP to be implemented, the school district may elect to assume liability for the device when used during school hours and assume responsibilities AT services to maintain the device.

OSERS, 1995 (Bachus letter)

- Eyeglasses are considered an AT device. When a child with a disability requires eyeglasses to receive FAPE and the child's IEP specifies that the child needs eyeglasses, they must be provided by the school district.

These clarifications assist the public agencies (school districts) to provide necessary equipment and services to children with disabilities.

Steps Toward Implementing Assistive Technology Services Within the Schools

To identify and implement AT devices and services for students with disabilities, the following steps should be taken:

Referral to Committee on Special Education

Any request for special education or related services, including AT, should be made in writing to the *Committee on Special Education* chairperson in the child's school district. This begins the process to provide the devices and services to help meet the child's education needs. The student's parent or guardian or a professional involved with his or her program can make a referral. Unlike Medicaid and private insurance, no medical need statement is necessary. The focus of AT here is educational: to give the child access to FAPE.

Assistive Technology Evaluation

A comprehensive evaluation of a student by a multidisciplinary team will determine the type and amount of special education and related service required for the student to receive FAPE. Assistive technology devices and services should be considered during the initial evaluation. If the school district personnel are not qualified to carry out an AT evaluation or if the parents disagree with their findings, parents have the right to request an independent evaluation. The school district is responsible for the cost of the evaluation(s). The AT specialists should collaborate with the student's IEP support team to identify appropriate AT solutions.

Assistive Technology in the Individualized Education Plan

The student's IEP must be written so that it includes any and all AT devices and services needed to meet educational goals in the least restrictive setting. The specific AT device, including all accessories and features should be identified, not just a general classification such as an AAC device. How it will be used to achieve these goals must be clearly stated: an estimate of the student's accomplishments in each domain, the conditions in which it will be used, and the criteria used to indicate the skill level. Specific training on a device before it can be used toward educational goals can be included as a related service.

Additional training needs are indicated if the student, the IEP team, or parents are not proficient in the use of the device to meet the student's educational goals. If the child requires the AT at home to benefit from its use, such arrangements should be included on the IEP.

Approval

After the IEP committee approves the devices and adds them to the student's IEP, the school district is required to purchase all listed AT services and devices.

The Interaction Between Medicaid, Private Insurance, and Public Education Funding

The primary source of AT funding is the child's school district when it is used to support the acquisition of educational goals. However, federal policy, as stated in IDEA, clearly indicates that other payers, such as private insurance or Medicaid, may be considered as a potential payment source for required services and devices, as long as the services and devices are available to the child at no cost to the family (34 CFR § 300–301[a] & [b]). Thus, if a school system wants to request payment through a private insurance company, they must ensure that the parents of the child will not incur a financial loss, including but are not limited to, the following:

- A decrease in available lifetime coverage or any other benefit under an insurance policy
- An increase in premiums under an insurance policy
- An out-of-pocket expense, such as the payment of a deductible amount incurred in filing a claim (45 Fed Reg 86, 390 [Dec. 30, 1990] restated 20 DELER 627–629 [Sept. 10, 1993])

Thus, the use of private insurance for AT devices and services must be strictly voluntary. When private insurance is tapped, the school district may pay any deductible fees or amounts not covered by the insurance company. This is to ensure that the devices are provided "at no cost to the parent."

Medicaid may also be considered in funding for school-based AT devices and services. Under Medicaid's EPSDT (early and period screening, diagnostic, and treatment) guidelines (see Appendix), all states must include OT, PT, speech therapy, and prosthetic devices to support the use of AT devices when seen as part of the "necessary supplies and equipment" in each service definition.

If Medicaid can be considered, there are tremendous opportunities for schools to shift the costs of many related services, including educationally necessary AT. Since 1986, Congress has enacted three laws that limit Medicaid's ability to refuse reimbursement to school districts for coverage for health services that are provided as special education or related services on a Medicaid-eligible child's IEP.

In Public Law 99-457, Congress acknowledged that funding systems other than the EHA or IDEA may be tapped to pay for the programs and services required by children with disabilities, and it identified Medicaid as one of the other financially responsible programs. The following year, Congress amended the Medicaid Act to parallel its statement in the P.L. 99-457 legislative history. The law now states:

> Nothing in this subchapter (Subchapter or Title XIX is Medicaid) shall be construed as prohibiting or restricting, or authorizing the Secretary to prohibit or restrict, payment under subsection (a) of this section for medical assistance for covered services furnished to a handicapped child because such services are included in the child's IEP established pursuant to part B of the IDEA, or furnished to a handicapped infant or toddler because such services are included in the child's IFSP adopted pursuant to part H of such Act [IDEA] (42 USC § 1396 b[c]).

Although written awkwardly as a "prohibition" or "restriction" of authority, this provision can be read as a foundation for Medicaid to provide reimbursement to schools for the costs of any related service, including assistive devices, that are otherwise included in the Medicaid program.

Procedurally, for schools to access Medicaid reimbursement, there must first be an agreement between the school district and Medicaid to have the school become a Medicaid provider. Second, there must be an exchange of information between the school and Medicaid to identify Medicaid-eligible children. Third, the school must follow Medicaid requirements for record keeping and billing.

If these conditions are met, Medicaid will become a provider of substantial reimbursement for the costs of a wide array of services to a substantial population of children with disabilities. For any service covered, the school district should be able to receive not less than 50% of the cost of the service, as compared with reimbursement for the same service at less than 10% under the IDEA.

Another legislative change in late 1989 further expanded Medicaid's in-school services reimbursement obligations. The law broadened the scope of covered services for children, making more services provided in school subject to potential Medicaid reimbursement. Specifically, the terms of the mandatory Medicaid service known as "early periodic screening, diagnosis, and treatment" or EPSDT were changed. (See the Appendix.) Effective April 1, 1990, children younger than 21 years of age are entitled to receive Medicaid reimbursement for services beyond the state Medicaid plan to include any service for which the federal government would provide reimbursement.

Read together, these legislative amendments enable school districts to obtain reimbursement for any related service on a child's IEP that "could" be reimbursed by the federal government, whether or not the service is otherwise listed on the state's Medicaid plan. Health screenings, OT, PT, speech therapy, audiology, counseling, nursing and health aide services, and a wide variety of AT devices are among the in-school services for which school reimbursement by Medicaid is now possible.

These changes in law represent a potentially significant means for school districts to shift the costs of their related services. In some states, millions of dollars are being added to school budgets because they are able to access Medicaid as a funding source.

At least one significant limitation does exist for children who are eligible for Medicaid and private insurance. Medicaid rules related to its status as payer of last resort, meaning that all third-party payers must be filled before Medicaid will pay, must be followed in the school setting. However, use of family insurance is severely limited by schools, as noted previously. Thus, a family with eligibility for Medicaid and insurance may not be able to have their child's school access Medicaid for the child's special education and related services needs.

Equipment ownership issues are one reason parents may choose Medicaid or private insurance funding for the needed devices or services. Any equipment purchased by the school district is the property of the district. This ownership issue may present difficulties as the child transitions to other schools within the district, when the child moves from one district to another, and when the child exits school entirely. Questions arise, such as whether the device moves with the child, even between school buildings. If a child moves to a new district, will the device move with him or her? What happens to the device when the child graduates or "ages out"? Ownership issues may also arise when use of the device in environments other than school is considered. By contrast, with Medicaid or insurance as the funding source, the family will own the device.

Successfully meeting the AT needs of students will require an ongoing examination of current systems and the development of new collaborative models. School districts are developing new policies concerning the use of AT devices and services. Some areas being considered include evaluation and use of devices, informed consent and the relationship of AT and other technology programs to the current curricula offered, and the development of long-range technology plans. In addition, because AT devices represent a significant investment in money and time, school districts need to develop tracking systems, make arrangements for maintenance and repair of devices, investigate sharing and loaning of equipment within single and multiple districts, and develop AT assessment teams to work with individual student teams.

SUMMARY

Funding is a critical issue. As stated in the outset of this chapter, without funding, nothing happens. Without funding, goals for functional improvement through the use of AT remain merely words on paper. The guidelines presented in this chapter are designed to provide therapists with the knowledge base needed to create appropriate funding requests and to enable access to AT for their clients.

STUDY QUESTIONS

1. Develop a checklist for your reports to Medicaid, including the needed information as well as "things to avoid," as they are described and presented in this chapter.
2. How do you decide which funding source is the best option when ordering an assistive technology device for a school-age child?
3. Differentiate between an *assistive technology device* and an *assistive technology service*.

REFERENCES

American Occupational Therapy Association (1991). Occupational therapy and assistive technology, Position Paper. *American Journal of Occupational Therapy, 45*, 1076.

Chandler, B. (1992). Special considerations I: Pediatrics. In J. Acquaviva (Ed.), *Effective documentation for occupational therapy* (p. 97).

Hehir, T. (1993). Letter to Seiler. USDOE Office of Special Education and Rehabilitative Services. Washington, DC.

Hehir, T. (1993). Letter to Moore. USDOE Office of Special Education and Rehabilitative Services. Washington, DC.

Hehir, T. (1993). Letter to Anonymous. USDOE Office of Special Education and Rehabilitative Services. Washington, DC.

Hehir, T. (1993). Letter to Bachus. USDOE Office of Special Education and Rehabilitative Services. Washington, DC.

Office of Special Education and Rehabilitative Services (1989). New federal support for technology services. *OSERS NEWS in print, 2*, 1.

RESNA (1992), *Assistive technology and the individualized education program*. Washington, DC: RESNA Press.

Schrag, J. (1990). Letter to Goodman. USDOE Office of Special Education and Rehabilitative Services. Washington, DC.

Schrag, J. (1991). Letter to Anonymous. USDOE Office of Special Education and Rehabilitative Services. Washington, DC.

U.S. Congress, *Public Law 94-142*, Education For All Handicapped Children Act of 1975.

U.S. Congress, *Public Law 100-406*, Technology Related Assistance for Individuals with Disabilities Act of 1988.

U.S. Congress, *Public Law 101-476*, Individuals with Disabilities Act of 1990.

Other Resources

There are two principal resources for IDEA information. These resources are required reading for a solid understanding of the IDEA and to remain current in this quickly changing field.

The *Individuals with Disabilities Education Law Reporter* (IDELR, formerly called the *Education for the Handicapped Law Reporter*) is the most comprehensive resource available. It is a multivolume reporter published every 2 weeks by the LRP Publishing Co., (215) 784-0860. It contains a complete copy of all the applicable federal laws and rules. It reports interpretive and enforcement materials issued by three U.S. Department of Education offices that administer and oversee the IDEA: Office of Civil Rights, the Office of Special Education Programs, and the Office of the Assistant Secretary for Special Education and Rehabilitation Services. The IDELR also provides the full text of selected state level administrative decisions and many federal court opinions.

The second recourse is a compilation of all final state administrative decisions involving special education. The state government (or a private publisher) may publish all final administrative decisions issued by the state Commissioner of Education in regard to IDEA (and other) issues. If published, these decisions will be available by subscription and are likely to be found in the government or legal documents sections of university or public libraries. Titles of these decisions may be "Opinions of the Commissioner of Education" or "Education Department Reports." Unfortunately, this compilation may not be available in all states.

Federal Medicaid Definitions of Primary Services Under Which Assistive Devices May Fall

EARLY AND PERIODIC SCREENING, DIAGNOSTIC, AND TREATMENT SERVICES

All states are required to provide early and periodic screening, diagnostic, and treatment (EPSDT) services. The broadest of all Medicaid services, EPSDT's goal is to implement the public health policies of prevention and early intervention to prevent, delay the onset of, slow the course of, or minimize the severity of disabilities. It is applicable to all Medicaid recipients in every state from birth through 21 years of age.

States are required to provide *inter alia*, periodic screening and evaluations consisting of age-appropriate developmental assessments that address gross and fine motor development, strength, balance, locomotion, eye-hand coordination, communication and language skills development, and self-help and self-care skills. They also must provide comprehensive, unclothed physical examinations.

The goal of these assessments, evaluations, and examinations is to determine whether the child has any impairments for which treatment services are appropriate. The standard is whether the child's functioning does nor does not match expectations for other children of the same age. If any impairments are identified, further diagnostic procedures will follow. The "T" of EPSDT requires the state Medicaid program to make available to the child all services available on the federal government's list of Medicaid mandatory-or-optional services to correct or ameliorate those impairments. As a result, children in every state must be able to access home health care services, durable medical equipment, prosthetic devices, occupational therapy services, physical therapy services, rehabilitative services, and as needed, skilled nursing facility services and ICF/MR-DD facility services. Each of these services is described below.

Another EPSDT characteristic is that medical need for services is the only permitted criterion for eligibility. State-imposed annual or other periodic limits on the number of therapy sessions, for example, do not apply to EPSDT recipients. Specifically with regard to assistive devices, state-imposed limits on the frequency with which certain devices can be replaced, (e.g., once per

5 years) will not apply to EPSDT. As long as the device does not meet the child's current medical needs, it can be replaced, regardless of when it was acquired.

HOME HEALTH CARE SERVICES

Home health care services are required by Congress to be a part of each state's Medicaid program, and the federal Medicaid regulations define home health care services to require the provision of "medical supplies, equipment and appliances suitable for use in the home." (42 USC § 1396a[a][10][a]; §1396 a[a][10][D]; 42 CFR § 440.70)

As a required service, home health care, and by extension, durable medical equipment, must be made available to all Medicaid beneficiaries, both children and adults. The only express limitation on access to this service is that beneficiaries reside in a home, which is defined to exclude hospitals, nursing facilities, and intensive care facilities.

All home health care services are provided on the basis of a physician's order as part of a written plan of care, and are reviewed every 60 days. Under these rules, a physician may request an OT or PT to conduct an evaluation and recommend the beneficiary receive an assistive device to address an identified need. Medicaid will pay for that device if prescribed for the beneficiary's use by the physician and if it meets additional state-by-state rules related to durable medical equipment.

DURABLE MEDICAL EQUIPMENT

Although it is a required component of home health care services, there is no further federal Medicaid definition of durable medical equipment. However, many state Medicaid programs have their own definitions, and therapists must determine whether they exist. In general, durable medical equipment has been defined to have four characteristics:

1. Can withstand repeated use
2. Is primarily used for medical purposes
3. Is generally not useful to a person in the absence of illness or injury
4. Is appropriate for use in the home

These criteria do not generally create funding barriers for many assistive devices, and they have been applied to provide coverage and funding for a wide array of assistive devices, including, but not limited to, the following:

- Bath and shower chairs and other bath and shower safety equipment
- Client lifts
- Stair glides
- Mobility devices
- Environmental control units
- Augmentative communication devices

- Seat-lift chairs
- Hearing aids
- Glucometers and talking glucometers

However, in some states and for some types of devices, the second and third criteria of the definition will cause funding problems.

The second criterion, that the device is primarily used for medical purposes, should be satisfied because the device is being requested to improve, restore, or prevent the deterioration of a beneficiary's functional abilities, all of which are medical purposes. Those effects are purposes or goals shared by all forms of occupational and physical therapy. The differences are in method, not purpose or goal, between services designed to strengthen the body's ability to perform functions in an unaided manner, and the provision of a device to support, supplement, or substitute for the body's residual functional abilities.

This criterion sometimes becomes a problem when Medicaid programs make judgments about the task for which a device will be used, instead of the intended role of the device as an aid to allow the beneficiary to perform a specific task in a more "typical manner" (i.e., as would a person without disabilities).

This barrier frequently is applied to augmentative communication devices. Rather than looking at the device as a supplement or substitute for the beneficiary's ability to communicate expressively, Medicaid may view the content or context of the communication as part of the funding determination. Medicaid will decide there is no need for the device because, for example, the beneficiary has no (other) unmet medical needs, the beneficiary is able to communicate with caregivers without it, or a child beneficiary will use the device in school or other nonmedical settings. All of these "rationales" are inappropriate and should be pursued further through additional communication with Medicaid staff or through appeal.

The third criterion, that the device is generally not useful to a person in the absence of illness or injury, can also be problematic. A device may be denied because it is used by the general public. The therapist must be sure to specify why a device, such as an augmentative communication device or environmental control unit, will be used by the beneficiary in a special way. Consider, for example, that for the person with severe muscular sclerosis an air conditioner or environmental control unit used to control appliances and other household items could make the difference between the ability to remain at home and the need for hospitalization or nursing home care. For the general public, the air conditioner is at most a convenience.

Other devices can be described as having dual uses (i.e., uses by the general public and specific uses by people with disabilities). A laptop computer used as part of an AAC device is one example. Some Medicaid programs address these issues by making specific references to this equipment or by providing a means for exceptions to the general rules to be requested.

In some Medicaid programs, exceptions are not available. In those states, consideration of funding for the devices under a different service, such as prosthetic devices, or directly under PT or OT, or contact with professional advocacy resources will be required to get past these barriers.

The fourth criterion, that the device be appropriate for use in the home, is rarely an issue. Most assistive devices are intended for use in the home or are portable and thereby able to be used in any setting.

OCCUPATIONAL AND PHYSICAL THERAPY SERVICES

Therapy services can be a source of coverage and funding for assistive devices, but therapists must first identify the manner in which these services are covered and whether the beneficiary meets the relevant criteria for access to that service.

The federal Medicaid regulations define OT or PT as follows:

Occupational Therapy means services prescribed by a physician and provided by or under the direction of an occupational therapist. *It includes any necessary supplies or equipment* (42 CFR § 440.110[b]).

Physical Therapy means services prescribed by a physician and provided to a recipient by or under the direction of a qualified physical therapist. *It includes any necessary supplies and equipment* (42 CFR § 440.110[a]).

Medicaid funding for assistive devices under OT and PT is based on the final sentence of the two definitions: "It includes any necessary supplies and equipment." Documentation to support funding for assistive devices will require proof that the device is "necessary to delivery occupational [or physical] therapy services" to the Medicaid beneficiary.

In many states, OT and PT services are further defined to include services related to the recommendation and fabrication of assistive devices. These references, while not uniformly included in state manuals or lists of procedure codes, provide a direct means for therapists to be paid for their services related to assistive device evaluation, recommendation, design, and fabrication. However, for Medicaid to pay for the devices, there must be a direct reference to how equipment is covered. In general, OTs should try to state that equipment is either an item of durable medical equipment or a prosthetic device, in addition to being equipment necessary to deliver OT or PT to the Medicaid beneficiary.

PROSTHETIC DEVICES

Prosthetic devices are one of the most common of the optional services provided by Medicaid programs throughout the country. They are required to be provided to beneficiaries younger than 21 years of age and are available to adults independent of their residential setting wherever states have elected to include them in their Medicaid plans.

Prosthetic devices are defined by the federal Medicaid regulations as follows:

Replacement, corrective, or supportive devices prescribed by a physician or other licensed practitioner of the healing arts within the scope of his practice as defined by State law to —

(1) artificially replace a missing portion of the body;
(2) prevent or correct physical deformity or malfunction; or
(3) support a weak or deformed portion of the body.
(4) CFR § 440.120[c])

This definition addresses a wide range of devices. Artificial limbs, artificial larynxes, white canes, braces, splints, car seats, and orthotic appliances are all within its scope. Augmentative communication devices other than electrolarynxes are also included: Prosthetic devices are the second most common Medicaid service into which AAC devices are classified, after durable medical equipment.

Documentation to support funding of a device, equipment, or appliance as a prosthetic device will require proof that the item will match the roles as defined previously. In addition to its direct application to many types of assistive devices, the definition of prosthetic devices has two particular uses: It can serve as a funding source for devices that fail to meet the definition of durable medical equipment and for devices needed by nursing facility and ICF/MR-DD facility residents.

REHABILITATIVE SERVICES

Rehabilitative services are also an optional service under the Medicaid program. "Rehabilitative services" is the general term used to describe OT and PT services that are a required part of the services available to nursing facility and ICF/MR-DD facility residents.

Rehabilitative services are defined by the federal Medicaid regulations to include the following:

Any medical or remedial services recommended by a physician or other licensed practitioner of the healing arts, within the scope of his practice under State law, for maximum reduction of physical or mental disability and restoration of a recipient to his best possible functional level (42 CFR § 440.130[d]).

In some states, rehabilitative services are the service in which OT and PT services are located. In other states, this service is targeted to rehabilitative services for substance abuse or mental health impairments.

One of the most important characteristics of the rehabilitative services definition is its statement of intent regarding the degree of functional improvement expected: "maximum reduction of physical or mental disability" and "restoration of a recipient to his best possible functional level." While these goals are consistent with the professional standards governing OT and PT and are consistent with the benefits to be conveyed by assistive devices, this goal is not expressly stated in any of the other Medicaid services that will cover assistive devices. In any state that uses rehabilitative services as the category of service under which OT or PT is provided, these goals must be included into all the recommendations and funding justifications provided to Medicaid: for example, "This device is required to enable the beneficiary to achieve his or her greatest reduction in physical disability." Another example is, This device is required to enable the beneficiary to achieve his or her best possible functional level."

SERVICES TO RESIDENTS OF NURSING FACILITIES AND INTERMEDIATE CARE FACILITIES FOR PEOPLE WITH MENTAL RETARDATION AND DEVELOPMENTAL DISABILITIES

Medicaid beneficiaries who reside in nursing facilities and ICF/MR who require assistive devices have a broad foundation of Medicaid regulations to support their requests.

The Medicaid regulations state that residents of nursing facilities

must receive the necessary nursing, medical and psychological services *to attain and maintain the highest possible mental and physical functional status, as defined by the comprehensive assessment and plan of care* (42 CFR § 483.25).

The regulations also require facilities to provide an environment that will promote "maintenance or enhancement of each resident's quality of life" (42 CFR § 483.15). Residents are given the right to choose activities, set their own schedules, and interact with others, both inside and outside of the facility, consistent with their individual interests. To achieve those functional goals, nursing facilities must provide assistive devices and services to people who require them.

Other nursing facility regulations directly protect residents' functional abilities. For example, the facility must provide services that ensure that residents maintain their highest level of physical functioning, including their ability to "use speech, language, or other functional communication systems"; their ability to transfer and ambulate; their range of motion; and their psychosocial functioning. Specifically, facilities must ensure that residents do not become withdrawn, angry, or depressed, which are definite risks if a person is not able to express his or her thoughts or feelings, sit comfortably, or get around independently.

To meet all of these requirements, facilities must provide the devices and services that are identified as needed by a comprehensive assessment. The devices that should be considered for nursing facility residents who may need them to achieve the goals described previously include augmentative communication devices, manual and powered mobility devices, specialized seating devices, prosthetic devices, and orthotic appliances. The OT and PT services required to conduct needed evaluations, recommend devices, aid in set up, customization, and training also are included in the regulations, as are other forms of "specialized rehabilitation service," such as speech-language pathology services.

The Medicaid regulations for ICF/MR facilities also impose standards for comprehensive assessment and plans of care and services. Of greatest importance, these facilities must provide "active treatment," which is defined as follows:

> A continuous . . . program, which includes aggressive, consistent implementation of a program of specialized and generic training, treatment, health services and related services . . . that is directed toward
> (i) the acquisition of the behaviors necessary for the client to function with as much self determination and independence as possible; and
> (ii) the prevention or deceleration of regression or loss of current optimal functional status.
> (42 CFR § 483.440[a])

To meet residents' needs, ICF/MR facilities are specifically directed to furnish, maintain in good repair, and teach clients to use and make informed choices about the use of communication aids, braces, and other devices identified as needed. In addition, the facilities must "identify mechanical supports, if needed to achieve proper body position, balance and alignment." Residents also must spend a major portion of each waking day out of bed, moving around by various methods and devices whenever possible.

One important benefit of assistive devices that is of particular importance to people residing in ICF/MR facilities is their ability to create new opportunities for their users. Among those new opportunities is the possibility of discharge to a less restrictive community-based setting. Independent communication and mobility, appropriate seating and positioning, and control over one's physical environment often are stated as prerequisite to life outside of institutional settings. Facilities must provide all the devices and services required for a resident to be discharged to the community.

INDEX

A "t" following a page number indicates a table; an "f"
indicates a figure.

241